THE FINAL SEASON

The

FINAL
SEASON

The Perseverance of
Pat Summitt

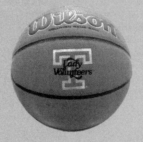

MARIA M. CORNELIUS

Foreword by
Candace Parker

THE UNIVERSITY OF TENNESSEE PRESS
Knoxville

Title page image: The Lady Vols logo is affixed to the team's official Wilson basketball.
Page vi image: © PMR photos.

Library of Congress Cataloging-in-Publication Data

Names: Cornelius, Maria M., author.
Title: The final season : the perseverance of Pat Summitt / Maria M. Cornelius.
Description: Knoxville : The University of Tennessee Press, [2016] | Includes index.
Identifiers: LCCN 2016009421 | ISBN 9781621903932
Subjects: LCSH: Summitt, Pat Head, 1952- | Basketball coaches—
United States—Biography. | Lady Volunteers (Basketball team) |
Alzheimer's disease—Patients—Biography.
Classification: LCC GV884.S86 C67 2016 | DDC 796.323092—dc23
LC record available at http://lccn.loc.gov/2016009421

Dedicated to my mother, Rosalie.
And Fido, my forever muse.

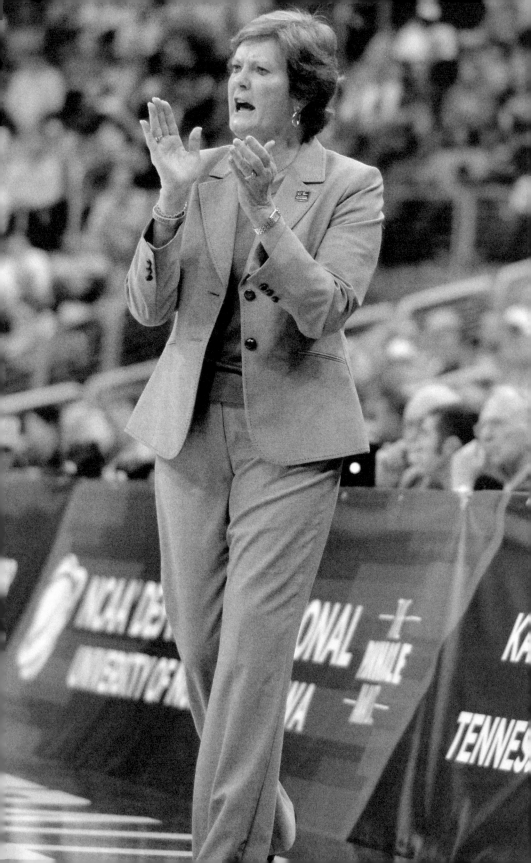

Pat Summitt
(1952–2016)

CONTENTS

ILLUSTRATIONS

FOREWORD

Pat Summitt is the strongest person I know. Coach's influence on my life has been instrumental in who I am as a basketball player, and more importantly, as a person. Her resume speaks for itself—1,098 wins and eight national championships and establishing the University of Tennessee Lady Vols as arguably the premier women's athletics program in the nation. But that only scratches the surface of her true accomplishments.

What sets her apart is her passion for the game, the development of people and the formation of lasting relationships. Coach is the most driven, dependable, strict yet fair, and honest person I know. Her recipe for success is the emphasis on the journey rather than the destination. The journey involves passion and people. She has always surrounded herself with quality people for whom she cares deeply. Her life is proof that consistent effort produces results. Winning games and succeeding in life is the reward.

It's hard to decipher in which way Coach has impacted me the most. She lives her own advice, rebounds from setbacks, always remains humble in success, positively adapts to the inevitability of change, and demands the best in herself and others. The lessons and stories are endless. But the lessons I was taught on the court always carried over outside the lines as well.

Pat Summitt's coaching was about defense and rebounding—the two things you can control no matter what. I had a tendency to stand on the perimeter and not crash the boards for offensive rebounds at times. Practices consisted of Coach screaming, "Parker! Rebound!" followed by the infamous

Author's note: The forewords were written prior to the death of Pat Summitt. The words will always resonate.

blue-eyed glare. My stubbornness often resulted in the entire team running sprints. Eventually, I figured out the importance of what she was preaching. Not only did my game greatly improve, but I also became a force on the boards and gained more possessions for my team. Her rebounding message taught me to overcome adversity, give myself additional opportunities, and try even harder the next time. Live in the moment. Control what you can, and do not spend time worrying about what you can't.

She was always there for me in good times and bad. Offering hugs after winning national championships, surgery, tough losses, and during family struggles, she was always supporting and loving. Her impact has trickled down to the way I parent my daughter, Lailaa.

In 2011, I received a phone call that I never anticipated. Pat shared with me her recent diagnosis of dementia, Alzheimer's type. My first thought was: She doesn't deserve this! As I stand by her while she takes on her toughest opponent, I see the qualities that produced a championship career—fight, determination, desire, focus—directed at conquering this disease for herself and unselfishly, for others. Who knew years ago that her impact would reach further then women's basketball? Through this illness she will do what she's always done: FIGHT and help others.

Maria M. Cornelius has been following and writing about Lady Vol basketball and Coach Summitt for 18 years. In *The Final Season: The Perseverance of Pat Summitt*, readers will gain insight into Pat the Coach and Pat the Person as seen through the eyes of the people she touched. Maria also captures the challenges and experiences of Pat's historical final season with the Lady Vols. This story needs to be told and shared.

Pat Summitt's impact is synonymous with wins and losses, but her legacy stands through her perseverance and character. Years removed from the last time I put on a Lady Vol uniform, I still hear her strong voice in my head, guiding me through my pro basketball career and life.

Candace Parker
Lady Vol, 2004–2008

FOREWORD

As someone who has been involved in women's basketball for 20 years, I have interviewed and encountered some of the biggest names in the industry. But none have reverberated and touched hearts like Pat Summitt.

Prior to following my passion and becoming a sportswriter, I was a marketing executive. I met some of the most inspirational giants to ever grace the earth: Tony Robbins, John Maxwell, and the like. But when it comes to women's sports and women in general, no one has been able to inspire like Summitt. She has been a tour de force that the game has never seen, and will certainly not see again. While the growth of women's basketball has slowly risen from the doldrums of national afterthought to more of a fixture in America's sports consciousness over the past few decades, none of this would be possible without Pat. She is truly the catalyst and Godmother of this game that we all dearly love. Her genius is second to none.

Summitt nurtured this wonderful game as if it were her child, she taught us all many lessons along the way, and she made sure to give us sustenance, too. She gave us all the "glare" if we needed it, and most importantly, she always put the game first. Everything Summitt did was advantageous, whether it was for her players, her fans, or the industry as a whole. Her avuncular character never allowed personal views to skew her interpretation of what was most important: growing the game that she treasured and nurturing young girls into exceptional women.

When it comes to children, you teach them lessons. Sometimes you discipline them, but you never hinder or stunt their growth. You show them love with a hug, then maybe you show tough love with a glare, but you are always giving love. Pat was always teaching us lessons, all the while never compromising her principles to win basketball games—and she's the greatest winner of all time. Without Pat, there is nothing. She got in the industry when it was relatively unknown and generating miniscule amounts of money for its coaches and teachers; however, that didn't deter her from pursuing the passion for the game that fueled her. Many contemporaries could learn a lot from this living legend.

Former players laud her, associates praise her, and everyone adores her, which speaks volumes of Summitt as an individual. So if anyone ever asks, "How can we grow women's basketball?" The answer is quite simple: Not only should we continue to "Back Pat"; we must also "Follow Pat." Follow her ways, follow her principles, follow her leadership, and most importantly, follow her integrity. That's how we can not only continue to grow this beautiful game, but also how we can back Pat and honor her legacy.

The woman who authored this book, Maria M. Cornelius, is someone who, in her own way, is like the lady she's writing about. In my time as a sportswriter and editor, I have never come across someone who embodied such veracity as Maria. Like Summitt, she is a woman of strength, high character, and fierce determination. She is a fighter and has a very incandescent soul. Growing up in the South, all Maria knew how to do was work hard—for everything. And with that dedication, she has continued to rise to success as a writer. But most importantly, she's an even better person.

When Maria was diagnosed in 2012 with her own life-threatening disease of breast cancer, she, like Summitt, didn't cower, wilt, or ask for pity. It was almost as if she channeled her inner Summitt and said emphatically, "I'm going to kick cancer's butt." She had a few scares along the way but has been cancer-free for nearly four years now.

Not to do too much reminiscing, but I met Maria in 2011 while covering the Dayton Regional in the women's NCAA basketball tourney. And from that moment until now we have become not just colleagues but true friends. In this very fickle industry, it is very hard, if not rare, to meet someone with whom you have great synergy and true friendship. In life, you hear the axiom about friends: "Find one good friend, you are fortunate." Well, I'm truly fortunate, because Maria is someone that I'm honored to call not only a friend, but also truly a great human being, and a true, altruistic ambassador for women's basketball.

When I think of Maria and this exceptional piece she's authored, I harken to a quote by Summitt that not only describes Maria, but also embodies Summitt's long-lasting message to all of us: "You can't always be the strongest or most talented or most gifted person in the room, but you can be the most competitive." Pat Summitt is not just a basketball name on a storied timeline; she is the embodiment of a life of excellence. Enjoy this book—it's one of the best works about Summitt that you will ever read.

In closing, PAT simply means, "Principled; Admired; and truly the heart of Tennessee."

Mike Robinson
Editor, *SB Nation's Swish Appeal*
Atlanta, Georgia

THE FINAL SEASON

PROLOGUE

started covering the Lady Vols in 1998. What began as filling in when needed at the *Knoxville News Sentinel* became a full-time job in 2004 for *InsideTennessee*. In 2013, just before securing my book contract with The University of Tennessee Press, I took a position as a writer/editor with Moxley Carmichael, the premier public relations and communications firm in East Tennessee. Cynthia Moxley, a seasoned journalist and communicator, founded the company in 1992. Her husband, Alan Carmichael, became president of the firm in 1998. They understood my need to keep writing on the side—especially about sports.

The column below, titled "Cover to Cover," initially ran in an early 2012 issue of *InsideTennessee*. It was republished on *InsideTennessee*'s website on April 19, 2012, the same day Pat Summitt announced her retirement, and it is repeated here as an introduction to this book. Some passages in the book also are from my final season coverage of Pat Summitt, especially the game summaries. This book is the result of my front-row seat to that final season and the subsequent multiple interviews with the people who were closest to Summitt.

While writing this book, I learned that my mother had been diagnosed with Alzheimer's disease. It narrowed my focus even more to finish it. Pat Summitt would be proud. And a portion of every sale will go to the Pat Summitt Foundation.

COVER TO COVER

The first time I called Pat Summitt, I made her mad. True story.

It was 1998, and her team had become celebrities. Led by the three "Meeks"—Chamique Holdsclaw, Tamika Catchings, and Semeka Randall—the group made news on and off the court. In February of that year, the team was undefeated and playing a delightful brand of high-octane basketball that packed the arena. It was also one season after the 1997 Cinderella season, which was memorialized forever by HBO. The Lady Vols lost 10 games that year and still managed to win a national title in Cincinnati by beating Notre Dame in the semifinal and Old Dominion in the championship game.

The program hosted a black tie film premiere of the HBO documentary at the Tennessee Theatre in downtown Knoxville with guests arriving in stretch limousines. This gala event occurred during the 1998 season upon the release of the film that winter. In addition, Pat Summitt had a book coming out called "Reach for the Summit," which outlined her principles for success. That needed to be reported, too. And there was still a season to cover with home and away games that chewed up the time of the Lady Vols beat writer for the local paper. That was how I came to work late one afternoon in February and ended up calling Summitt.

At the time I was the night editor for the *Knoxville News Sentinel* on the news side after spending several years as a police and court reporter. That desk position meant I arrived to work with little time before the first deadline, since the early edition of the paper headed across the state and needed to get to the trucks before the evening had actually ended.

The sports department had been tipped off that Pat Summitt was going to be on the cover of *Sports Illustrated*, and the news side wanted it on page one of the next day's paper. A photo image of the cover was set to arrive soon. Meanwhile, the sports side was covered up with, well, sports. The beat writer had games to attend and was often on the road trying to handle daily coverage of the team, and news kept popping up that had nothing to do with the court. So the sports side asked the news side for help ferreting out the *Sports Illustrated* story. It was early in the last week of February, a Tuesday if my memory is correct. The issue with Summitt on the cover would be for the following Monday, March 2.

I arrived to work right as these discussions were taking place between the departments. The news reporters were filing their stories that had been gathered that day and would be headed home soon. I was a desk editor that funneled story copy through the night production process so a paper would be delivered the next morning, but I had not stopped writing when called upon to help and welcomed any chance to do so. I also was a lifelong sports fan. That meant I had barely gotten to my desk before I was selected to get the Pat Summitt cover story and get it fast. I had less than two hours to verify the story with *SI*, interview someone with the magazine, get Summitt's reaction, and file the story to meet deadline.

This was in the 1990s when news reporters called people directly. We didn't go through a layer of spokespeople. Several prominent officeholders didn't even have a media contact. If I needed the police chief or sheriff or a judge or the district attorney, I called their office. If it was after hours, I called them at home. This was also before security and access tightened so much—the pre-9/11 world—and newspaper reporters walked directly into offices for interviews. I had been on the night police beat for years and would take doughnuts (no, it's not a cliché) and coffee to the detectives' office and sit and chat about major crime cases they were working for follow-up stories, such as homicides and armed robbers on hold-up sprees across the city and county.

So, I wouldn't think anything about picking up the phone and calling Pat Summitt's office to determine her whereabouts. I was aware of Deborah Jennings, her longtime media relations chief—she is recognized as the best in the business—and the fact I didn't call her to set up the interview wasn't an attempt to circumvent the process. I just wasn't aware of the process. That wasn't how the news side operated at the paper.

I also had very little time with the front-page editor saving a big space for the photo, which had now arrived from *Sports Illustrated* and depicted the classic Summitt stare. The clock was ticking, and my supervisor reminded me that I needed to reach Summitt soon. So I made the first call. She wasn't there. If she had been, I would have dashed over to her office to interview her there. I left a message. I waited maybe 10 minutes. I called back.

I wasn't being rude. Again, this was normal for the news side. We were used to calling officeholders, appointed officials, mayors, governors, etc.

Persistence was standard procedure. Plus, I was running out of time. The business day was coming to a close and university staff members would be leaving to go home. This was before cellphones had taken over communication. People needed to be reached by landlines. The window of contact would soon close for the day.

I repeated this callback process. About the fourth or fifth time, I detected that the secretary answering the phone was getting a tad peeved. Again, this doesn't cause a news reporter to flinch. I just remained polite, explained it was very important for a page one story, and reiterated that I really needed to reach Summitt. A few minutes after the last attempt, my desk phone rang. The person on the other end sounded a lot more peeved than the secretary. It was Summitt.

When the coach confirmed she was speaking to me, a clipped voice said, "What can I do for you, Miss Cornelius?" The emphasis was on Miss and my last name, and the tone was controlled seething. Apparently, she had been very busy that afternoon. I have since learned that Summitt scheduled her day down to the minute. Her calendar was a color-coded chart of places to be, people to see, and phone calls to take. To say the least, my name didn't appear on her calendar that day.

The secretary, knowing Summitt was very busy, had apparently been alarmed enough by my repeated phone calls to track down Summitt and get her to call me. The conversation was probably something along the lines of "this reporter won't leave me alone and you really need to call her back now." As could be expected, Summitt likes to know why people are calling her—especially ones she does not know. That is what the media relations staff do in all arenas, whether sports or politics: they determine who you are and what you want, how much time you need, and what the topic will be. But I didn't have time for that. I had a front-page editor asking me every five minutes if that gaping hole in the cover story was going to be filled.

I had never met Summitt. In fact, we had never spoken, not even on the phone. I was a little startled by her tone and thought that the *SI* cover photo had certainly pegged her. Of course, I now know I had panicked her secretary and Summitt had been pulled out of a previously scheduled meeting of some importance to deal with some pesky reporter. I thanked her for the call back, said she would be on the cover of *Sports Illustrated*, described it, and said I needed her reaction. The cover was a big deal. Female athletes had been on the cover, but she would be the first female coach to grace that page.

The phone went silent. I wondered if we had been disconnected. After a few seconds, a soft voice said, "Can you repeat that?" I did, including the title words "Wizard of Knoxville," a play on John Wooden being the "Wizard of Westwood" while at UCLA. "Wow," Summitt said, still with a quiet voice. Clearly, this had stunned her in a good way. Of course, I needed more than one word for my story. So after she got over the shock, she answered my questions in the tone that is so familiar now—straightforward and engaging. She also credited the players and said any honor she got was shared with them. I have since learned this is common with Summitt, too. She will rarely take credit for anything.

My memories go back to that day with the news in December 2011 when Summitt and Duke Coach Mike Krzyzewski had been selected as *Sports Illustrated*'s Sportswoman and Sportsman of the Year. This was Summitt's reaction: "Obviously, this is a tremendous honor. I am so privileged to share it with such a great coach in Mike Krzyzewski. During our careers, we have both been fortunate to work with so many talented student-athletes who were driven to excel both on and off the court. For me, this recognition is a direct reflection of the outstanding young women who have worn the orange and white Lady Vol jersey of the University of Tennessee; the coaching staffs I have worked with throughout my career and the supportive administration at UT." Nearly 14 years had passed between covers for Summitt, but she was essentially unchanged. The credit went to everyone.

Time Inc. Sports Group editor Terry McDonell said, "The voices of those who have been inspired by Pat Summitt and Mike Krzyzewski echo from everywhere and will continue for decades. What they have achieved through their coaching and, more importantly, their teaching places them among history's transcendent figures. It is an honor to now include them in the select group of Sportsmen and Sportswomen."

SI senior writer Alexander Wolff had this to say about the selection: "More than that—so much more—are the roads each has traveled over the course of careers that can be measured in Presidents Met on White House visits with Team (four in her case, three in his). For their endurance, for their adaptability, for their genius for hatching from adversity even more success, and for their willingness to take up causes beyond the comfort of their own campuses—indeed, for modeling what it means to be public diplomats as well as great coaches—we honor them as *SI*'s 2011 Sportswoman and Sportsman of the Year."

Both are the winningest coaches ever in NCAA Division I men's and women's basketball, and both were recognized for that achievement. Krzyzewski reached that pinnacle in December 2011, and Summitt did so in 2005. Both are still adding to their win totals and continue to be admired for how they conduct their lives off the court.

In Summitt's case, she revealed in August 2011 that she had been diagnosed with early onset dementia and would continue to coach. She and her son, Tyler, have set up The Pat Summitt Foundation to raise awareness of the disease and funds to find a cure. The announcement sparked a "We Back Pat" campaign at the University of Tennessee that was adopted by the SEC for an entire week with men's and women's teams using home games in January as a chance to promote the foundation.

Since that first cover in 1998, Summitt has continued to win. The program's sixth national title came at the end of the 1998 season with a perfect 39–0 record, sparking another book with co-writer Sally Jenkins, *Raise the Roof*. Two more championship trophies were added in 2007 and 2008. The 2011–12 team, with four true seniors trying to reach their first Final Four, wanted to add another trophy to the display case in the basketball office. That is always the goal at Tennessee, but Summitt's medical diagnosis added a greater sense of urgency and purpose.

Summitt has handled having dementia the way she approaches everything in her life–head-on, no "pity party," and in the open. Her mother, Hazel Head, probably liked the 2011 cover over the 1998 one. She remarked in 1998 that she wished the magazine had selected a photo of her daughter that showed her smiling. She got her wish with the 2011 issue, which depicted Summitt, basketball in hand, standing beside an also smiling Krzyzewski.

I have one more Summitt story about that 1998 season.

The SEC Tournament was in Columbus, Georgia, that year, and Summitt's first book, *Reach for the Summit*, was about to be released. The newspaper received an advance copy, and I was asked to review it and interview Summitt. I had also handled the HBO documentary debut in Knoxville and ended up in Kansas City to cover the fans at the Final Four in 1998 for the news side of the paper. Eventually I became the go-to for Lady Vol basketball stories that occurred off the court, and that is ultimately how I ended up at *InsideTennessee*.

But in 1998, I was just a person with a ticket to the SEC Tournament and an advance copy of Summitt's book in my hand. I saw her sitting in the stands with her assistants and walked over to introduce myself. This was the last week of February, just days after I had persistently called her office about the *SI* cover, which was starting to reach newsstands. Fans were bringing items over for her to autograph.

I sat in a seat to the side of her and pulled out the book. She looked stunned and said, "Where did you get that?" The book was weeks away from release to the public, so a seemingly random person sitting down and pulling out a copy was understandably surprising. I explained who I was and why I had the book, and once again her tone changed, and she smiled. I then saw the Summitt everyone else meeting her in person had described—warm, engaging, gracious.

I asked if I could interview her about the book later—I had just gotten it, so I had not read it yet—and she smiled and said, "Call my secretary to set it up."

We both laughed.

THE ROSTER

Briana Bass, player, final season

Vicki Baugh, player, final season

Angie Bjorklund, former player

Cierra Burdick, player, final season

Andraya Carter, final recruit

Joan Cronan, women's athletics director

Mickie DeMoss, assistant coach

Bashaara Graves, final recruit

Isabelle Harrison, player, final season

Debby Jennings, chief of media relations

Glory Johnson, player, final season

Jasmine Jones, final recruit

Dean Lockwood, assistant coach

Alicia Manning, player, final season

Heather Mason, strength and conditioning coach

Ariel Massengale, player, final season

Jenny Moshak, chief of sports medicine

Candace Parker, former player

Meighan Simmons, player, final season

Taber Spani, player, final season

Shekinna Stricklen, player, final season

Pat Summitt, head coach

Meshia Thomas, police officer and Summitt's security guard

Holly Warlick, associate head coach

Kamiko Williams, player, final season

1

THE ANNOUNCEMENT

Vicki Baugh wasn't a typical college student. She wasn't typical, period. The player called "grandma" by her teammates was raised in Sacramento, California, by her grandparents, Barbara and Calvin Baugh, and she oozed an old soul personality. The fifth-year player didn't have social media accounts while in college, so she didn't know big news was breaking that day. "I've always been called the grandma of the team," Baugh said. "I got Facebook super late. I am not into Twitter. I finally got an Instagram. I am not big on social media, so I actually had no idea."

It was a sun-splashed August day in East Tennessee. Fall semester classes were barely underway and full-scale court workouts were several weeks away, so the players were scattered across campus and the surrounding area. A group text message reached most of them that morning about a mandatory team meeting early in the afternoon. "We knew it was something serious. We don't usually have meetings before the season like that," said Glory Johnson, a senior and native Knoxvillian.

Pat Summitt and her chief of media relations, Debby Jennings, had prepared a video the day before of the head coach announcing that she had early onset dementia. It was to be posted to the Lady Vols website and disseminated to the media as soon as the team meeting ended August, 23, 2011. But the news leaked on the Internet about two hours before the meeting, and while some players weren't yet aware of it, others were already getting calls asking what was wrong with Summitt. "I went straight to the basketball office, and they were furious because it had leaked out," Jenny Moshak said. "What they were upset about is that Pat really wanted to tell the team herself. The team was receiving texts and tweets before they got to the office."

Moshak, the longtime chief of sports medicine for Summitt, became aware of the diagnosis the day before when she got a call from the basketball office. Moshak, who can explain a player's injury from a decade ago with total recall, struggles to remember the exact details of how she learned about Summitt. Assistant Coach Dean Lockwood had the same reaction when asked about the day he found out. Details remain fuzzy, an indication of how traumatic the news was for the staff, as the brain scrambles to protect the heart.

"Somebody called me from the basketball office and said they wanted me to hear it from them and then they asked me to get ahold of Heather, because they couldn't get ahold of Heather," Moshak said. Heather Mason served as the team's strength and conditioning coach and had been handselected by Summitt, who called her the toughest coach on campus.

"I called, and Heather was driving her car, and I told her," said Moshak, who first directed Mason to pull over. "That is when we both broke down. It hit us both very, very hard. When the basketball office called—and for the life of me I can't remember who it was—I went into information mode. You get bad or crisis news and then you've got to disseminate the information to the proper people. After I did that, that is when I broke down. Then it was about what it was about. That was rough. Heather and I talked a long time on the phone."

On the day of the announcement, Moshak was in another meeting when she got the text about the team gathering. She left immediately and headed to the basketball office. Nearly everyone was there except Alicia Manning, who was tracked down and arrived a few minutes later. Summitt's son, Tyler Summitt, was present, as was Joan Cronan, the acting UT athletics director and the longtime women's athletics director before the men's and women's athletics departments were combined. It was an off day for the team, and the upperclassmen had received a text message instructing them to make sure the younger players got there, as the meeting was mandatory. The players knew something was amiss based on the faces of the staff. The fact the news was spreading across the Internet only added to the anxiety.

"Pat wasn't as upset as the other coaches," Moshak said. "Pat was Pat. When I walked in the door, several of the coaches were pacing. They weren't real happy. The players were hearing about it, and they were trying to get the players there as fast as they could. I was standing there and the national Alzheimer's office called the main office. You could see it come over the caller ID, and they did not pick it up. All they wanted to focus on was telling the team."

"That was a day you can't forget," Taber Spani said. "They called an impromptu team meeting after people got out of classes. They held it in the film room of the office. Everyone was kind of on pins and needles because you didn't really know exactly what was going on and what was going to be said." From Lee's Summit, Missouri, sharpshooter Taber Spani was in orange for one reason: she wanted to play for who she considered to be the greatest basketball coach of all time. Spani respected Summitt, but she also adored her as a coach, person, and mother. She is very close to her parents, Gary and Stacey Spani—they also favored Tennessee because of Summitt, especially after their recruiting tour allowed them one-on-one access to head coaches—but Summitt was basically a second mother to Spani.

"It was right about 1:15. I had just gotten out of class," Meighan Simmons remembers. "I knew there was something going on because it wasn't the same. The coaches' office, everybody just seemed so reserved. There wasn't much conversation. Normally in the coaches' office everybody is jolly and communicating with one another. We were scared because we didn't know what the meeting was about. But we didn't think it had anything to do with Pat."

Simmons idolized Summitt and still does. The slender scorer from Cibolo, Texas, was another player who wore orange simply because of Summitt. She was surprised by the text message, because the first week of class was usually pretty quiet as far as basketball duties were concerned. Meanwhile, Glory Johnson and fellow senior Shekinna Stricklen had just returned from China the previous evening after winning the gold medal at the World University Games as members of USA Women's Basketball. Summitt, who met the pair at the airport, had been awaiting their return to tell the entire team together. Cierra Burdick was in the Thornton Center studying when she learned of the team meeting. She had spent most of the summer training and playing with the U19 team for USA Basketball at the 2011 World Championships in Puerto Montt, Chile, so she had officially been a Lady Vol for just a few days. The freshman caught a ride to the arena on one of the golf carts used by the Athletics Department to scoot personnel and players across campus.

"We had our struggles, so I am thinking this is another meeting about how we pull together," Baugh said. Baugh was on the national championship team in 2008. The Lady Vols had reached the Elite Eight in 2011 but had fallen short of the Final Four. In Knoxville, the season is deemed unsuccessful if Tennessee isn't one of the last four teams standing. In 2011, the season ended with a particularly desultory performance against Notre Dame—an underappreciated team at that time that was on its way to being a Final Four fixture. As Baugh walked across campus, she thought Summitt wanted to set the tone early for the 2011–12 season. "And then I noticed the demeanor of the coaches," Baugh continued. "It was something that was different, something seriously wrong. I knew the news was very important that was coming. And then when she laid it on us. . . ."

Summitt didn't waste any time getting to the point.

"I remember when Pat said the words," Assistant Coach Dean Lockwood said. "She was very open, very direct and honest. She said, 'I want you to hear this from me. I have been diagnosed with dementia.' There was this stunned silence for several seconds. Every eye was on Pat and then slowly, 15 to 20 seconds, people start to look down, tear up, some looked away. Some put their head down in their hands. It was a very, very somber meeting."

Some of the players had family experience with Alzheimer's. Others were unclear as to what exactly Summitt had just said. "I remember being really confused because at the time I didn't even know what dementia was," Burdick said. "Everybody was making a really big deal out of it, and I didn't understand why. I didn't understand the significance of it. The biggest thing I remember from that meeting is Pat saying, 'We're going to be alright.'"

"When I heard that, all I could think of was bad," Simmons said. "I didn't completely know what it was. I just knew there was something wrong. It was so shocking that you didn't know what to say. All you can do is sit there." Some of the players had already heard the news because of its earlier release on the Internet, which moved rapidly across social media. "I don't know if they necessarily believed it until they heard it from Pat," Moshak said. "Their parents were hearing it, and they were starting to contact them."

"I remember being in that room and Pat, in typical Pat style, just went right to the point and said what she was dealing with and how tough it had been and how she had come to grips with it," Spani said. "Right away she went to how she was going to battle it and how she would always be there for her team. I remember her making a joke: 'No, I haven't forgotten any of your names.' Pat broke the ice a little bit with that."

The fifth-year player who had endured two major knee surgeries was the one who finally broke the silence of the players. "It was Vicki Baugh who spoke first," Lockwood said. "She said, 'Pat, we've got your back and whatever you need from us.'" Her words became a battle cry and touched off a "We Back Pat" campaign that continues to this day. "I just let her know immediately she had been there for me through everything—personal family issues and on the court and dealing with my injuries—so the first thing that came to my mind was you have my back and we have yours," Baugh said. The rallying cry reached Summitt's heart immediately. "It really touched me. I was all but having tears," Summitt said. "I love her. What a great leader."

Summitt did all that she could to ease the players' minds and emphasize that the focus was on their well-being. "There wasn't a dry eye in the room except for hers," Burdick said. "She kept saying, 'We're going to stay strong,' and 'We're going to get through this.' She was the one going through all of it, but she was also the strongest one in the room." The news was staggering, especially to Spani, who would repeatedly break down crying in the days afterwards. "I remember walking out of that meeting very emotional. I basically came to Tennessee to play for Coach Summitt, and playing two years under her, I developed this amazing relationship with her and just like that things changed," Spani said.

"I remember her saying, 'I am here for you guys. And we're going to take this and I don't want anything to be about me.' It was incredible how selfless she was in the whole thing. The entire Lady Vol nation and really the whole sports nation for those first few days, everyone was glued on this announcement, and she was turning it into a call for us to rise up and fight for each other. It ended up being something that brought us closer. We wanted to give everything we had, not only for the program, but for her. She was so selfless and didn't make it about her. You can't forget something like that."

The impact of Summitt had long been known, but it was underscored the day she told the team she had Alzheimer's disease. The topic dominated local and national news and was accompanied by an outpouring of support. And while Summitt's news seemed to envelop the sport, the Lady Vols became a very insular team as they prepared to embark on a season that came without a how-to manual. "A lot of tears. A lot of rallying. A lot of motivation. A lot of support. A lot of hugs," Lockwood said. "Tried to keep a sense of normalcy, as well."

That would become a season-long theme.

_2_

SPRING AND SUMMER 2011

Dean Lockwood was the third assistant coach on the staff to know Pat Summitt had dementia. Holly Warlick and Mickie DeMoss knew about a week earlier, because Lockwood was on vacation in his home state of Michigan and was sometimes out of the reach of wireless devices. The two other assistants opted to alert him after he returned to Knoxville.

May is one of the few quiet months for basketball coaches. The players are finishing exams and getting ready to go home for a few weeks before summer school starts. The head coach's basketball camps are in June—all hands are on deck for those, including the players'—and July is a month-long, cross-country journey to evaluate recruits, with international trips added if Lady Vol prospects are playing in USA Basketball world championships events. So May is the one month when coaches take vacations and, in Warlick's case, the month of her annual motorcycle ride with former Lady Vol Nikki Caldwell, the head coach at LSU, to raise awareness and funds for breast cancer research.

In 2011, Summitt used May to travel to the Mayo Clinic with her son, Tyler. She knew something was wrong, though there were valid explanations. Rheumatoid arthritis had taken its toll on her joints, and the medications to alleviate the pain and symptoms could cause memory loss and confusion. The staff and players had noticed changes in Summitt, though nobody thought it rose to the level of dementia. DeMoss had returned to Tennessee for the 2010–11 season after stints at Kentucky and Texas. DeMoss had been by Summitt's side from 1985 to 2003. The time away from Tennessee gave her a different perspective on Summitt, and she noticed some changes.

"She was just quieter," DeMoss said. "She seemed a little bit more detached from the program. She wasn't constantly talking and coaching. That is just not Pat. That was not the Pat that I knew. I was very concerned. But I didn't know. You certainly don't want to jump to conclusions. It wasn't just one day or one moment. It was a process." While DeMoss wasn't overly alarmed, she did push for Summitt to get a thorough health assessment at season's end.

Examinations at the Mayo Clinic confirmed that Summitt had early onset dementia, a diagnosis she resisted before coming to terms with it over the summer. Tyler immediately took charge of the situation in terms of a medical plan back home and restructuring of finances. Immediately after the trip to the Mayo Clinic, Summitt went to Destin, Florida, for the SEC annual meetings. June and July were filled with summer basketball camps and recruiting, and then the reality of the diagnosis hit her in August. Summitt retreated to her darkened bedroom for several days, and it took Tyler breaking down to get her to her feet.

Lockwood returned to Knoxville from vacation and learned of the diagnosis. He still struggles to recall the details of how he found out. "Here's the thing. A lot of things I can have crystal clarity about, but that isn't one of them," Lockwood said. "Pat went to the Mayo Clinic in the spring. We were noticing things. She had decided it's time to go and something's not right. She went and came back. I don't know who she told first and when, but she laid low for a while. She didn't just come back and say, 'Here is what happened.' When I came back is when I knew for sure. It was later in May when I actually knew it had been diagnosed."

Warlick was among the first to know. She went to Summitt's house soon after the return from the Mayo Clinic. "I suspected something. I noticed very subtle things. You explain it by being tired, and I forget stuff," Warlick said. "But to hear her say what she said . . . you are talking about this person who had been sharp and on her game all her life. You find out she has this disease. She was crying. We were crying. We were at her house on her back porch. It was so surreal. She was telling us about the testing." Summitt was hosting an event that day, so after telling Warlick, she had to immediately get ready for guests. "We ended up going over to the pool house," Warlick said. "Pat said, 'I can use it to my advantage.' She said, 'I can have anything I want to drink. And if someone says, 'Pat, you're drinking too much,' I can say, 'I forgot. I have dementia.'"

The coaches closed ranks as they determined how to proceed. Debby Jennings, of course, was told. She had been a trusted confidant of Summitt's for 35 years. Joan Cronan, the interim athletics director at that time, and UT-Knoxville Chancellor Jimmy Cheek were notified in August, a few days before the team was told. Summitt went into the August meeting with longtime lawyer Robert B. Barnett, who had forewarned the head coach that the school could ask for her resignation. Instead, Cronan and Cheek cried, vowed to help Summitt as much as they could, and told her she would remain coach for as long as she wanted to do so. Summitt expressed a desire to coach for three more seasons, if possible.

"Your first thing—and I am wired this way; I was raised this way—but you protect people in your program," Lockwood said. "This place has always been like that. Pat has always run it like that. She brought people in her circle and you did things together and confided in one another. It is more like a family than just colleagues." Lockwood coached on the men's side at Tennessee with stints at Northwood University in Michigan, Central Michigan, and Saginaw Valley State University. His admiration and respect for Summitt had always run deep. He worked her camps, and while Lockwood was a Vols assistant coach at Tennessee from 1986 to 1991, he would watch her practices and takes notes. Summitt was a coaching colleague and friend to Lockwood, and he returned to Knoxville in 2004 for one reason: the chance to work for her. Now, he had to ponder the sea change he knew was coming.

"I was just very sad and certainly thought of the implications. How is this going to impact her? Will she be OK? My dad had dementia in the late years of his life. How soon will we see another turn? I thought about her coaching and how much she loved coaching and how this would, quite honestly, shorten the time she had left to coach. I wasn't dwelling on them by the hour, but those things were in my head. And really it came back to this: 'What is best for Pat? What do we need to do to protect Pat and this program?'"

The basketball community is a close-knit and insular one. Coaches, especially ones like Summitt who have been in the game so long and won multiple national titles, are closely scrutinized by their colleagues. Lockwood heard from one of those coaches about two weeks after the 2010–11 season ended. He declined to identify the coach but said her intentions were those of concern: "There was a Division I coach that loved Pat. Just respected Pat to the nth degree. Read every book that she's done. Read every clinic note that she could get her hands on. She studies Pat. Every time a game is on, she watches. And she called me that spring about two weeks after the season was over and she said, 'I don't mean to pry. Is Pat OK?' I said, 'What makes you ask?' She said, 'I've just noticed there's a difference. She is not quite the Pat I have seen. There is just something that is different. She is just not the same. I just hope she is OK.'" The staff had been asked about Summitt during that season, too. Tara VanDerveer, the longtime coach at Stanford, had inquired about her colleague. Those who had known Summitt well—or like the coach, had watched her so closely—noticed changes, although nobody thought it was as serious as Alzheimer's.

Summitt was one of the game's trailblazers and a major reason TV contracts became commonplace and women's basketball coaches became well compensated. She was well liked and respected, but the staff also knew there were some among their ranks who would try to exploit her diagnosis, especially in recruiting. Some coaches were jealous of Summitt and resented her popularity and ability to reel in top recruits, and a vulnerable Summitt would be an opportunity for them to pounce. It would become brutal once the news was officially released later that summer, so the coaches tightened the circle around Summitt on the road while they still had control. It wasn't easy, however. Summitt is popular at any gym she enters. Coaches want to talk to her. Fans want autographs. Photographers turn their lenses in her direction.

That started with the summer recruiting circuit. Coaches sit on bleachers for hours in gyms that sometimes lack air conditioning. It is very cozy and also a time for coaches to chat informally, away from the daily pressures and demands of the season. "That summer we made an extra effort to circle around her if people were trying to get too close," Lockwood said. "People just want to be around Pat, and she is so welcoming. We were a little bit of a buffer. We didn't want people who were prying and trying to find out more." Former players and those close to Summitt penetrated the buffer. The rest were kept from getting direct access to her. "We wanted to keep them at bay," Lockwood said. "There were other people we felt like we kind of needed to have our radar and antenna up [around], and we circled up around her. We were aware of that at the onset."

The staff knew the news would rock the sport. The first step was for the coaches to adjust to a different but still quite capable Summitt: they had to get through a vital recruiting period unscathed. The second step was to tell the Tennessee administration: that went very well with Cronan and Cheek. The third step was to tell the team. The final step was to announce it publicly.

When the players walked out of the basketball offices on August 23, 2011, they were about to embark on a basketball season like no other.

3

THE CLASS OF 2012

Pat Summitt sat on the couch, an empty dinner plate in front of her on the coffee table. Just six weeks after announcing her illness of early onset dementia, Summitt was in the living room of Lady Vol recruit Andraya Carter on a home visit.

"Where are your dogs?" Summitt asked. The head coach knew Carter's family had dogs. She made it a point to know the minute details about the high school players who were offered scholarships to Tennessee. When told the dogs were in a back room so as to not disturb the guests—Associate Head Coach Holly Warlick also made the trip—Summitt said to let the dogs loose. A snorting pug and a large black Labrador romped down the hallway like a runaway freight train and went straight to Summitt. She laughed and showered them with affection while Andraya's mother marveled at the down-to-Earth woman that she was meeting for the first time.

Jessica Lhamon had long known about Summitt. Her first-born child had vowed to play for the Lady Vols since elementary school. But with three other school-aged children at home in Alli, Zoey, and Curt, Tyke Lhamon took the unofficial visits to Knoxville with his stepdaughter, Andraya, to see the Lady Vols play. Andraya chatted with Summitt and the staff after those games, as did Tyke.

Summitt also came to Georgia to watch Andraya play at Buford High School, so she had spoken to the highly successful coach, Gene Durden, whom Andraya credits with helping her get ready to play at Tennessee. But Summitt wasn't allowed by NCAA rules to make contact with parents on those school trips, so Jessica had yet to meet the iconic head coach until that fall day in 2011. "We saw her when she came to Buford to watch games, but we never talked to her there," Tyke said.

Jessica remembers well the first time Summitt came to see her youngest daughter play. When Summitt arrived at a high school gym, it was an event. Local media documented her presence. Fans swarmed for photos and autographs. In this case it was Buford, a short distance from Andraya's home in Flowery Branch. Jessica, who knew Andraya's heart was set on wearing orange, had borne her first child while in high school and raised her with the assistance of Andraya's paternal grandmother, the late Gloria Carter. She married Tyke when Andraya was 4 years old, and he became a big part of her quest to become a Lady Vol.

Jessica was nervous—something that continued throughout college, as she could rarely watch Andraya play basketball and instead paced the concourse if present or went to a back room of her home if on television—because she knew how much her daughter wanted to impress Summitt. Andraya is a gifted athlete of sinewy build and with a standing vertical leap of 30.5 inches, a measurement that so surprised testers they made her jump three times to verify it. The 5'9" guard didn't score a lot when Summitt visited, but Andraya played lockdown defense and got on the boards, that leaping ability on full display.

Andraya was worried after the game, because while she had scored in other games, she didn't tally many points when Summitt was there. Jessica was also fretting, fearing the head coach would not be impressed, but Tyke knew better: his daughter's motor made her perfect for Summitt's trapping and full-court defense. Indeed, Summitt spoke to Durden after the game and left no doubt she wanted Andraya to be a Lady Vol. That message got delivered to Andraya, who committed to Tennessee as a 10th grader in 2010 and never wavered from that decision.

The day the news broke about Summitt's dementia diagnosis, Jessica called her daughter, who was at school. Andraya had already heard. "It was a short conversation because she wanted to know who to get in touch with to get the word out that her mind wasn't going to change," Jessica said. "She literally said, 'OK.' I said, 'Are you OK with that?' She asked, 'Is Pat going to be a part of the program?' And I said yes, and she said that was all she needed to know. Her loyalty was to the program and Pat and Holly. She said, 'Mom, who do we need to call?'"

Andraya let it be known via social and traditional media that her commitment was firm. She didn't want other coaches to start trying to recruit her away from Tennessee, a legitimate consideration because the Lady Vol coaches were also worried the commitment class would get cannibalized less than three months before the early signing period for high school seniors in November 2011. Like clockwork, Jessica received four calls from numbers she didn't recognize within hours of Summitt's medical news being made public. She is not certain of who was on the other end because she didn't answer, but the calls stopped as soon as Andraya publicly reiterated her commitment. "It didn't happen before, and after that day it didn't happen again," Jessica said.

Summitt needed that loyalty in the weeks after her announcement, one that rocked the national sports community, as the iconic coach seemed invincible. She got it from Andraya and two other recruits from the high school class of 2012, Bashaara Graves and Jasmine Jones. They kept their verbal commitments and inked letters of intent that November to play for Tennessee after making a pact to stay together. It would be the last class that Summitt signed.

Andraya understood loyalty. Three months before Summitt's announcement, the rising high school senior tore the ACL in her left knee in a pickup game after school while lunging for a steal. The family knew they had to tell Tennessee about the injury, a serious one with a lengthy rehab that would cost Andraya most of her senior season in high school. "We had to call Pat and tell her that Andraya was injured," Jessica said. "She was like, 'OK, how can we help? Just so you know she is family. She is part of the program. Nothing changes.'"

After Summitt's news was made public, the coaches went calling on the new recruits. Andraya was thrilled to welcome Summitt into her home, a tidy, well-appointed house in a quiet subdivision about 45 miles from Atlanta. Summitt, Warlick, and the family gathered in the den and sat on couches or the floor. "We are pretty laid-back," Jessica said. "I don't cook, so I wasn't going to cook a meal. Tyke cooks, but he was at work, so we got takeout." Tyke, a supervisor at the Rohrer Corp. in Buford, arrived home in time for the visit. He played baseball for Ohio State, so he was well aware of big-time athletics and the recruiting process. Coaches are used to having to woo parents as much as players, but Tyke told the coaches they only had to focus on Andraya. "You don't have to sell me on Tennessee," Tyke said. "Andraya is the decision-maker."

Summitt and Warlick presented Tennessee's case, one that focused on Lady Vol tradition, commitment to academics—every player that completed her eligibility at Tennessee graduated under Summitt—and expectations. "We ate and Pat said, 'What are your questions that you have for us?' And I was like, 'Do we have questions, Tyke?'" Jessica said. Tyke said Jessica asked a few "normal, mom questions," but the visit was relaxed, and Summitt seemed the same to him. "I was completely at ease. I said, 'You've answered all my questions.'"

He was at work when he learned about Summitt's disease via a news alert on his phone, and he knew immediately that her career would be truncated. "I expected she would step down. I thought it might be a year or two down the road," he said. "It was sad news, and I was disappointed that Andraya wasn't going to have Pat as the head coach, but I knew that Pat would still be around. She had done it for so long, and I knew she would not just walk away." Summitt and Warlick had gone to Buford High School earlier in the day to visit with Andraya and watch a knee rehab session before going to the house to meet the family. That led to the relaxed meal and Summitt's desire to let loose the dogs.

"We were sitting around and she said, 'I thought you had dogs,'" Jessica said. "And we said, 'We put them up because we didn't want them to jump on you.' Before I could finish the sentence, she said, 'Well, go get them!'"

The loves of Summitt's life, besides her son Tyler, were her dogs, Sadie and the late Sally Sue, both Golden retrievers. Warlick has Labrador retrievers. Hero, a large black lab that thinks he's a lap dog, immediately took to the coaches. "They loved the dogs, and the dogs loved them," Jessica said.

Andraya reiterated her firm commitment on the visit. The two other recruits had vowed to stay, too, but the Lady Vols coaches went calling, just to be certain and to show the mamas how much they wanted their daughters.

Several years later, one of those mamas, LaTrish Jones, settled into a chair in the lobby of the downtown Marriott in Knoxville. She was in town for a game during the 2013–14 season, as she so often was to see her daughter Jasmine play. Jones, a defensive stalwart for the Alabama women's basketball team in the 1990s—she played against Tennessee All-Americans Chamique Holdsclaw and Tamika Catchings—looked as if she could still take the court, her body tall and lean. When Tennessee and the Crimson Tide clashed, Jones would draw the All-Americans as her defensive assignments.

"Bless her heart," Summitt said with a smile.

LaTrish needs no history lessons when it comes to SEC women's basketball and Summitt; she had a vantage point from the court while playing for the Crimson Tide. "I knew at that time Pat Summitt was the greatest women's basketball coach in history," LaTrish said. "Obviously, as a female playing basketball in the South, I would want to play for Pat. I knew then Pat was the man, the woman in women's basketball."

LaTrish gave birth to Jasmine while still in high school, but that didn't deter her from becoming a college athlete. As a toddler, Jasmine played courtside during practices at Alabama, so she grew up to the rhythmic sounds of a gym and the colors of crimson and white. Despite the early indoctrination into Alabama, Jasmine's eyes turned towards the orange.

"Once I found out that my daughter was actually pretty good in basketball, I wanted nothing but the best for her," LaTrish said. "It was going to be her decision where to go, but in my mind, the best was Tennessee; regardless of if I went to Alabama, the best was Tennessee. Not UConn. Not Baylor. You can't get any better than Pat. Getting her ready for college, in my mind, if she's good enough for Tennessee, then she is good enough for anyone in the country. If Pat wants her, then she has arrived. Period."

Jasmine committed to Tennessee in the winter of 2011, three months before Summitt's diagnosis at the Mayo Clinic and six months before the news became public. LaTrish got a call that summer day from her daughter's coach at Bob Jones High School, and he broke the news about Summitt. "He told me, and I went online and I saw it online," LaTrish said. "I had another call on my phone, and it was Pat. She was leaving a message saying that she wanted to talk to me and Jasmine, so she was trying to get in touch with us before it really got out."

LaTrish's first reaction was one of compassion for Summitt. At the time, her grandmother was in the final stages of Alzheimer's. "Immediately I was sad. I knew what was coming," LaTrish said. "I also knew she had time. Her mind is always percolating. You just wouldn't think that would happen to someone who is always doing something." LaTrish's second action was to compose a speech about commitment to deliver to her daughter after school. "I let her know whatever she decides, I am with her, but I spoke to her about loyalty first and foremost," LaTrish said. As it turned out, LaTrish didn't need to summon any oratory persuasion. "She said she wanted to be a

Lady Vol, and it just made my day. It would have broken my heart even more if she said she wanted to switch schools. I didn't know if she just wanted to play for Pat or be a Lady Vol. Obviously, she wanted to be a Lady Vol. Being chosen by Pat was a big deal."

Summitt and Assistant Coach Dean Lockwood, who had been the primary recruiter, arrived for the home visit. The pair went to Jasmine's high school, and Summitt was, as always, well received when she entered. "I was out of town on work, and we flew in at the same time," LaTrish said. "They arrived at the school before I did. They watched practice. Pat signed autographs. Everyone loves her. They had to make the kids not pour into the gymnasium. When practice was over, they came to the house, and we went out to eat." What LaTrish remembers most about the visit is how normal it was. Summitt seemed like herself, engaging and at ease. "Nothing different than what we had seen before," she said.

Keinya Graves noticed the same thing when Summitt arrived in Clarksville, not far from Summitt's Tennessee hometown of Henrietta. Keinya's grandmother was diagnosed with dementia, also at a relatively young age, so she was familiar with the disease. "I found myself looking and watching and seeing how she was doing," Keinya said. The family decided to take the staff to a landmark restaurant in Clarksville called Johnny's Big Burger. "It is Bashaara's favorite restaurant in Clarksville," Keinya said. "Johnny's is basically a greasy spoon, and one of Bashaara's favorite things is a honey bun with ice cream. We were trying to get her [Summitt] to eat a honey bun with ice cream, and we knew she would not. She ate the ice cream off of the honey bun. We sat there and just talked. She seemed fine."

Bashaara wasn't fine the day Summitt's illness was announced. She was distraught and needed her mother. "Bashaara's high school coach told her, and she called me crying," Keinya said. "Her coach had told her after practice what was going on." Keinya was already on the way to the high school to pick up Bashaara after practice, so she reached her daughter quickly. "She needed a hug, and she needed someone to listen. I told her, 'It is going to be OK. Your future is going to be your future. We are going to make it regardless,'" Keinya said. "By the time we got home—we live not even 10 minutes away from the school—she had gotten a message from Andraya, and she had gotten a message from Jasmine. She was in her room, and she was talking to both of them. By the time Holly and Dean called her, she was good."

Keinya knew exactly what to ask Bashaara: the same thing she had during the recruiting process. "I asked her, 'Do you feel comfortable? What exactly do you want to do?' So when that came up, I put it the same way," Keinya said. "I was like, 'It is up to you. I don't have to play. You are the one who has to go. You are the one who has to feel comfortable in the situation once you get there. If you are not going to feel comfortable, you have to make this decision now, rather than waiting until you get there.'" Bashaara didn't need long to decide to stay and told her mother she was still headed to Knoxville. "I said, 'Are you OK?' And she said, 'Yeah, I talked to Draya. I talked to Jasmine. They're staying. I'm staying.' That was it."

The three players entered into Lady Vol lore that day. The trio said yes to Tennessee at a time when the program needed it most. Had the class of 2012 unraveled so soon after Summitt's announcement, it would have signaled serious cracks in the Lady Vols' storied foundation. The letter of intent documents—LOI in the game's parlance—that Carter, Graves, and Jones signed were the last ones in history to be affixed with Summitt's signature. "It's weird to think we were the last class to be signed by Coach Summitt," Carter said. "We talk about it sometimes. We mainly talk about how it was really cool that we all three stayed."

Keinya reacted the same way as the mothers of Jones and Carter. Her first thought was the well-being of Summitt. "At first we were more concerned about how she was doing, of course, and how it was affecting her before we were worrying about whether or not she would be coaching," said Keinya, who was able to talk to Summitt later that day after the announcement. "She reassured me that she was going to be around Bashaara. She didn't say exactly in what type of aspect, but she did reassure us that she would be around."

4

BASKETBALL BEGINS

One week after having their basketball lives forever altered, the Lady Vol players began to take the court again in preparation for the 2011–12 season. The NCAA allows limited workouts after classes begin and before the official start of practice, and players can work with the coaches in groups of up to four for two hours per week. They also have several hours per week as a team with the strength and conditioning staff. Since the sessions are limited to four players or less, they are often initially grouped by positions. In fall 2011, Vicki Baugh took the court with fellow post player Isabelle Harrison. (Glory Johnson had an additional week off since she had spent several weeks in August with USA Basketball.)

Harrison, a freshman, walked onto the court expecting basketball drills like the ones she had done all summer without the coaches present. She didn't expect to see the staff until October. Baugh had to explain to the newcomer that the coaches were now allowed on the court with players since fall semester had started. As a recruit, Harrison wasn't as heralded as her classmates Ariel Massengale and Cierra Burdick, who were high school All-Americans; however, it didn't take long for Pat Summitt to like what she saw from all three that first week. "They are not shy in the least," Summitt said. "They don't mind asking questions. Ariel, she has really stepped up and been a leader. And Cierra, same thing. If she doesn't know something, she's going to come over and ask. They just want to get things right. Izzy is impressive. She catches on very quickly."

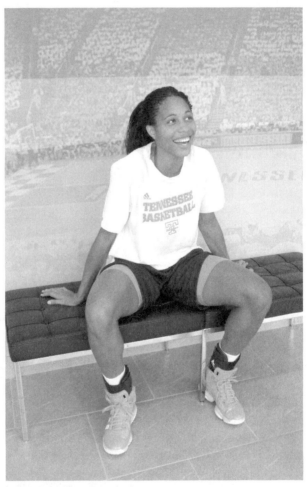

Isabelle "Izzy" Harrison always had a smile on her face. She was a freshman post player for the final season.

By her senior year, Harrison had developed into one of the best post players in the country—arguably the best interior player in that high school class as it turned out—proving that high school accolades and recruiting rankings can't measure the heart, determination, and hard work it takes to succeed in college. It was bittersweet for Harrison and her classmates: they arrived on Tennessee's campus in the summer, only to find out a few weeks later that their head coach had early onset dementia. Harrison, while just a freshman, knew every player had a heightened sense of responsibility to the program, because scrutiny would now be even more intense. "Everybody is going to be looking at us," Harrison said. "For one, because we're Tennessee. And for two, because of Pat's dementia."

After the news about Summitt broke on a Tuesday, a campaign, fueled by social media, encouraged people to wear orange. Burdick and Harrison grabbed a video camera to get reactions from students. "We were pretty much going around and asking students, 'What made you put on this orange today? What does Pat mean to you all? Why did you want to come out and show support today?'" Burdick said. "A lot of them said, 'Pat has done so much for the university, and we just want to show our respect for her.' Just to go around to complete strangers, athletes or not, and see how much respect they had for a woman they had never even met—that is tremendous. That just goes to show how much she truly has done for the game of women's basketball."

Summitt chatted with the media after that first workout session the same as she always did. During her career, she was one of the most accessible coaches to fans and media. She opened practice sessions to the public. She talked to the media after each one, and if needed, she did three one-on-one interviews with the local television stations. During those early workouts, Summitt still allowed access to the media—though Tennessee would change that policy when the 2011–12 season officially started—and she was always comfortable with the press, especially those who had been around the program for years. Summitt tried to overturn the decision to close practice—she wanted fans to be able to attend, as usual, when sessions were in the arena—but she was overruled by the Athletics Department administration.

In her typical fashion, Summitt was ready to take the spotlight off of her and place it on the players, though she was grateful for the outpouring of support. Katie Wynn, her longtime secretary, was in charge of compiling all of the emails and messages. "I appreciate all of it, but I've got to get ready and focus on the season, and that's what is up next," Summitt said. The Lady Vols and Vols share Pratt, which has a huge wall between the two courts that can be raised or lowered so either team can make use of the full facility or half of it. As the Vol basketball players left the weight room and crossed the court, they all patted Summitt on the back as they walked by.

Summitt nodded and smiled at the Vols while continuing to talk to the media. "It really has been very touching." Meanwhile, the players welcomed getting on the court after the tumultuous nature of the past week. "For myself—and I'll talk for even my teammates and my coaches and my trainers and my managers—I think the court is somewhat of a stress reliever," Burdick said. "And when we get in between these lines, it's like all of our worries go away, and it's just us and the ball and we're a team and a family. We don't have to worry about people coming and asking us what's going on. We get in between these lines, and we're cracking down to business."

Baugh and Johnson were on the court together for the second post workout with the coaches of the 2011–12 season. Both were entering their last year as a Lady Vol, and both had already earned bachelor's degrees and were enrolled as graduate students. Baugh was a fifth-year player because of multiple knee surgeries, a situation that ironically allowed her to be on Summitt's final team. Johnson was the best overall athlete that Summitt had ever recruited to play basketball. A state champion sprinter with eye-popping leaping ability, Johnson was a local product of Webb School of Knoxville, where she had been coached by former Lady Vol Shelley Sexton Collier.

Baugh remembers walking onto the court for that session not knowing what to expect. It was her first time to see Summitt with a whistle around her neck since the announcement. "We were nervous to talk to her," Baugh said.

Johnson sometimes irked Summitt with her tendency to make a flashy play instead of a fundamental one, such as going for a finger-roll layup at the front of the rim rather than using the backboard. Summitt's voice would boom across the court when that happened, and it didn't take long for Summitt to assert herself at that workout. "Glory did something, and she yelled at her, 'Use the glass. I'm not impressed,'" Baugh said. "We were like, 'OK, what are we doing? This is still Pat.'"

Meanwhile, Burdick had no past experiences of comparison when it came to Summitt at practice. "For me, it was just like the norm. Pat was my head coach," Burdick said. "There were times I got the stare, and Pat chewed me out in practice. I still remember the first time I got chewed out. I don't remember what I did. I do remember me being like, 'Jesus, well, that was it. That was what everybody talks about. I just got the wrath of Pat

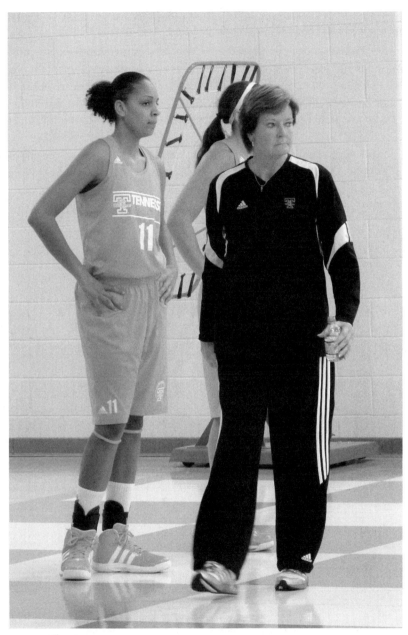

Cierra Burdick with Pat Summitt at practice. Burdick considered herself blessed to be given that one season with Summitt.

Summitt.' And I don't remember what I did. I was just so focused on what had just happened with her yelling at me."

Summitt is known for her withering stare and intimidating sideline presence, but her players also know her for a sarcastic sense of humor and biting wit. That approach set the players at ease immediately because Summitt made sure Alzheimer's became something she could laugh about with them. "Pat is a total jokester," Baugh said. "She joked with us, 'Maybe I'll forget that.' Or, 'Don't think I'm going to forget that.'"

Still, basketball is serious business at Tennessee. And a team of five seniors with a head coach whose future was uncertain wanted nothing more than to get to the Final Four, somewhere Tennessee hadn't been since 2008.

5

VICKI BAUGH

Candace Parker, one of the most decorated players in Tennessee history, predicted Vicki Baugh would be Tennessee's next All-American. A 6'4" forward, Baugh had a game very similar to Parker's with smooth interior skills, a fluid midrange jump shot, the ability to handle and pass the ball, and a competitor's heart. Baugh injured her knee in Tampa in 2008 during the national title game against Stanford on a beautiful drive to the basket; she completed the play despite shredding her ACL on the way to the rim.

Baugh, in excruciating pain and clutching her left knee, needed assistance from Jenny Moshak and Dean Lockwood to get off the court. The play happened directly in front of the Lady Vols' bench, and as Baugh hobbled off the floor, she pointed to the somewhat shell-shocked players and screamed, "Let's go, y'all! Let's go!" The moment galvanized Tennessee, which went on to win its eighth national title by utterly stymieing the scoring of Stanford. The Cardinals, picked by five of six national prognosticators to win because of its intricate and well-executed offense, didn't even reach 50 points.

"When you squeeze an orange, you get orange juice, because you get what's inside," Lockwood said a month after that April 8, 2008, game. "When you squeeze a human being, you get what's inside. At that moment, life and basketball were both squeezing Vicki. She suffers a devastating injury and yet in the midst of all that, she's concerned with not herself, not her injury, not get me to the locker room, she's concerned about our team."

Baugh returned for the 2008–09 season, but she tore her ACL again in February 2009 and missed the entire next season in 2009–10. The game that ended her season was against Oklahoma on February 2, 2009, in Oklahoma City, and it was memorable for another reason, too: with help from 6'6" Kelley Cain, and the stout defense of 6'3" forward Alex Fuller, the Lady Vols halted an NCAA record double-double streak by 6'4" Courtney Paris. The Sooners' senior center had posted 112 consecutive games with double figures in points and rebounds, a streak that started in December 2005 when Paris was a freshman. Paris grabbed 12 boards in the 80–70 win over Tennessee but tallied just nine points before fouling out with 41 seconds left in the game.

Summitt was particularly peeved after the loss because, in her view, the players had selectively followed the scouting report, especially with regard to the Sooners' Whitney Hand, who lit up the Lady Vols for 20 points and hit four shots from the three-point arc. So Summitt, who was sitting on 999 career wins, decided the players would scout the next opponent, Georgia. An out-of-conference loss to Oklahoma in February could be put in the rear-view mirror, but Georgia was a conference game, and the Lady Vols needed SEC wins. Letting players handle the scout was a risky move.

Summitt and I shared this exchange two days before the game:

The coaches are letting the team do a scouting report?

"I'm not *letting* them do it," Summitt said after a long pause.

So you're making them do it?

"Think about it," Summitt said. She then went on to outline the six to 12 hours the coaches invested in scouting reports per game and the 12 to 16 hours Betsy McAllister, the team's video coordinator that season, took to pull together film clips and condense them into a scouting report for the players and coaches. "And then we go out there and we don't know who the best three-point shooter is? And if they do, they're not committed to defending the best three-point shooter? After that game I was like, 'No! No!' Holly was at the end of her rope and rightfully so," Summitt said. "Because she had that scout, and she invested so much in it. So if they're going to have any against Georgia they have to do it themselves. Nobody went to film session with them."

It worked. Summitt's 1,000th win was delivered with a 73–43 decimation of the Lady Bulldogs in front of 16,058 fans on February 5, 2009. Baugh watched that game from the sideline—an MRI the day after the Oklahoma game confirmed a second ACL tear to her left knee. The injury came after she caught a lob pass, landed awkwardly and, yet again, completed the layup. It was late in the game, and Baugh was, once again, playing at her best. She had injured the lateral collateral ligament in the same knee on January 1, 2009, at a practice in New Jersey and had played sparingly for a month. She returned for the Oklahoma game and scored 11 points in 24 minutes, a tantalizing indication of how much better Tennessee was when she was on the court. "We're all heartbroken," Summitt said the day after the injury, her voice heavy with emotion. "She's such a great kid. She has worked hard. When you have one of those even the first time around it's like, 'Why me?' I can only imagine what she's thinking now."

Baugh underwent the major surgery and devoted herself to another grueling rehab. The 2008–09 squad was full of freshmen and one sophomore in Angie Bjorklund. Baugh and redshirt senior Alex Fuller, who also battled knee issues, were the team's leaders. When Baugh went out, a young team continued to crumble. Fuller did all she could, and Summitt recognized her as one of the best leaders to ever play at Tennessee, but a team that was "young-minded" in Fuller's estimation took its toll even on Fuller, who had migraines so bad that she once had to be hospitalized during that season because of the pain.

"A lot of people talk about this and that, but they don't know what our team went through," Baugh said. "I was one of the team leaders, and I couldn't play." Baugh played the 2010–11 season but had a third knee surgery after it ended to address a meniscus tear. The knee issues derailed what should have been a stellar career for Baugh, but those same knee issues also meant she was still in Knoxville for Summitt's final season. It was Baugh's words that launched a national campaign of support and led to "We Back Pat" shirts being worn by opposing teams.

Summitt needed Baugh that season. Baugh knew the program inside and out. She could mentor the young players, especially Izzy Harrison, the freshman post, and Baugh became a calming influence on the team. "Everybody listens to her," Summitt said. "Vicki is that kind of player, and she is that kind of person. She will draw people in. She will be the first to get somebody in the huddle and say, 'We've got to pick it up.'"

Baugh saw Summitt at her absolute best when the head coach led her team to its second consecutive national title in 2008. The Lady Vols won in

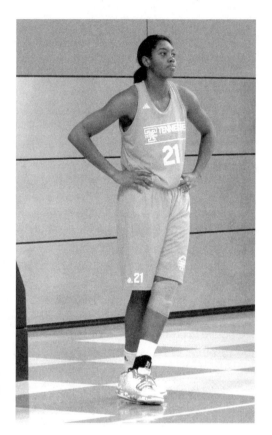

Vicki Baugh, shown on the baseline at Pratt Pavilion, would become the leader of a team that needed her wisdom and experience during Pat Summitt's final season.

2007 behind the leadership and rebounding of Nicky Anosike, the dominating play of Candace Parker, the defense of Alberta Auguste and the spunk and big shot capabilities of Shannon Bobbitt and Alexis Hornbuckle. Baugh joined that group of five for their farewell season—all five were drafted by the WNBA the day after winning a second national championship—and carved out a spot for herself despite being a freshman.

Entering the 2007–08 season, Summitt's biggest task was to keep her core five motivated and focused. Baugh had a daily view in practice and games of how Summitt challenged and forged another championship campaign. The 2008–09 season was an ordeal with the departure of five starters and with Baugh struggling to get back to form after having major knee surgery and then reinjuring the same knee. That season marked the debut of Glory Johnson and fellow freshmen Briana Bass, Alicia Manning, and Shekinna

Stricklen, a group that started their careers with one of the worst seasons in Lady Vol history and ended them by playing in Summitt's final game.

Baugh and Johnson became very close and ultimately ended their time in orange together. Playing for Summitt that final season forged team bonds that will never be severed. "The team became unbelievably close," Baugh

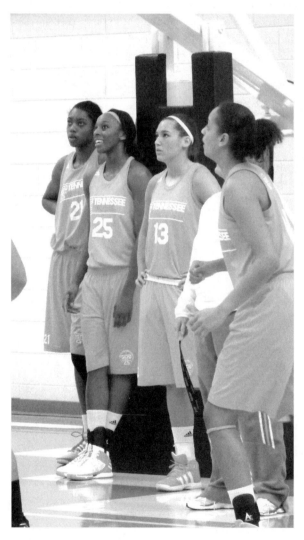

From left, Vicki Baugh, Glory Johnson, Taber Spani, and Cierra Burdick at practice in Pratt Pavilion.

said. "I started hanging out with Glory more. I ended up learning a lot about my teammates, learning a lot about myself as far as how I could push through things. I appreciated life. I grew as a person. It was rough but at the same time it was life changing for a lot of us. And I know Pat will love that."

Johnson knew the 2011–12 season would be a daily test of the team's will and resolve. "Your coach, a mother figure that you look up to and someone you care so deeply about, and you have to play the whole season knowing that she is sick," she said. "And knowing it's going to be in the media, and she's not going to have good days, and we have to be able to play through that and find ways to comfort her and our teammates . . . we're going to have to deal with it. We're going to have to figure out a way."

6

PRACTICE BEGINS

The Lady Vols form a circle before every practice at center court, whether in Thompson-Boling Arena, Pratt Pavilion, or any gym anywhere in the country. The shoes of each player, staff member, and coach touch the shoes of the person on either side, a symbolic way of closing the circle. The last game may be discussed. Or the previous practice. Announcements are made, such as meetings or reminders of team functions off the court. Dean Lockwood reads the quote of day. It is a routine that the players learn early, as do recruits. When high school players make visits to Tennessee on a day that practice is held, they join that circle before watching from the sidelines.

Meighan Simmons remembers forming a circle at the first official practice of the 2011–12 season on October 5, 2011. The team had been on the court for limited workouts—no more than two hours per week in late August and the month of September. But October signaled the start of the season, when a two-hour practice is considered a relatively short one. So many things still seemed the same: Pratt Pavilion, practice uniforms, the circle. But this season was very different for the second-year player.

"I will never forget the feeling of knowing that nothing was going to be the same," Simmons said. "It was heavy on my heart. Pat made such an impact on me my freshman year and built me into the basketball player that she wanted me to be and that she expected me to be. So knowing that she wasn't going to be able to interact with us as much or talk with us as much, it was heavy on me because I am so used to hearing that voice. And that voice is just so strong to the point that it becomes habitual in your head, where nobody else's voice matters. I will never forget that feeling of missing a big piece of me that I had carried with me my first year going into my second year, knowing that she wasn't going to be able to do as much."

Local media always covered the start of practice, and for this one, the national media arrived as well. Summitt always opened practice to the public—in fact, during her first head coach emeritus year the following season in 2012–13, she saw two longtime reporters sitting outside waiting for practice to end so interviews could be done. She stopped to chat, noting it was "ridiculous" that the reporters weren't allowed inside.

Summitt wanted practice open for the 2011–12 season, but the Tennessee administration overruled her shortly before the first exhibition game in November. The intent was to avoid any potentially embarrassing situations for Summitt, if she were having a bad day. But rather than show Summitt dealing with the disease on a daily basis, the cameras zeroed in on her during games and fixated on the coach if she appeared at all out of sync. The game footage distorted Summitt's final season and rarely looked anything like the still photos taken during the game that showed her engaged with players and coaches. It didn't capture her regular interviews during the season with media, none as feisty as her session before the NCAA Tournament in March 2012 when longtime New York Times reporter Jere Longman asked about her long-term plans. Summitt knew Longman, a respected writer, and her familiarity and comfort showed as she answered his questions.

The Knoxville media did have regular access to Summitt, and her illness became secondary to the coverage of the season. That wasn't always the case on the road, however, and one incident angered Summitt when a Tennessee newspaper columnist, despite knowing that she had been ill for 24 hours with a stomach virus, narrowed his piece to call attention to the devastating effects of dementia. She had a right to be upset; it was a distorted portrayal of Summitt at that point in the season.

When practice started that October, media members from print, television, radio, and Internet lined a side wall of Pratt Pavilion for the two-and-a-half-hour session with boom mics hovering overhead for the national media's audio needs. Robin Roberts of ABC-TV's *Good Morning America* and production crews from the network's news show *20/20* were in town for interviews with Summitt and to get video footage of the Tennessee head coach at work. Roberts, a former basketball player and cancer survivor, accurately portrayed both Summitt's disease and her status as head coach.

The scurrying of media members along the sidelines didn't faze the players. Summitt's policy of open practice had prepared her teams well for press coverage. "Being at Tennessee you're going to get a lot of attention, not only at the games but at practice," Baugh said. Summitt was either on the court or under the basket at practice and spoke to players one-on-one. Afterwards, she also spoke to the media. It had been just six weeks since Summitt had publicized her diagnosis, and she and the staff wanted to restore a sense of normalcy for the players.

"A lot of the aftershock of Pat's news had been done, because that was revealed in August," Dean Lockwood said. "It was back to business as usual. We had a season that was starting. We had a team to coach. It was new water that we were swimming through, figuratively speaking, for all of us. Until you go through it, you really don't know what you're going to encounter or what adjustments and changes you'll have to make. That day, I remember, it was practice as usual."

Returning to the rhythms of basketball was a relief to all involved with the program. The first week of full practice, along with intense preseason conditioning and weightlifting sessions, meant the players' days were filled—early morning workouts, classes, afternoon basketball practice, homework, and sleep: a routine that stays on repeat during the season.

Tennessee also hosted a batch of recruits on the second weekend of October, including the class of 2012 commits who stuck to their verbal agreements and signed scholarship papers in November 2011—Andraya Carter, Bashaara Graves, and Jasmine Jones. They were on official visits as high school seniors "I think it speaks volume to the kind of character that the three young ladies have," Mickie DeMoss said. "When Pat announced her diagnosis, they could have very well bailed on us."

High school juniors Kaela Davis and Diamond DeShields made unofficial visits that same weekend, the difference being schools pay for official visits while the recruits are responsible for the costs of unofficial ones. Davis and DeShields, who both are from Georgia, were fairly frequent visitors to campus, and the Lady Vols had long been recruiting both players.

The staff knew that publicizing Summitt's condition could affect recruiting, a cutthroat process under any circumstances. Tennessee had long been

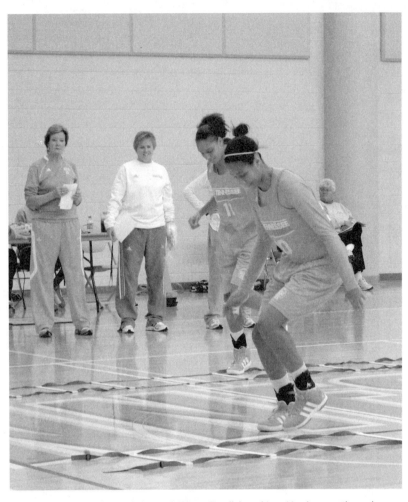

Pat Summitt and Holly Warlick watch Cierra Burdick and Izzy Harrison go through footwork agility drills on the court during preseason.

successful and long been subjected to negative recruiting by rival schools wanting to knock the Lady Vols off their perch. Tennessee also ran a clean program in a sport that has become beset with the unethical tactics that infect men's recruiting. The NCAA, burdened with trying to police football and men's basketball, has basically turned a blind eye to the escalating shenanigans in women's basketball.

Rival recruiters, in what is best described as predatory behavior, seized on Summitt's condition to create doubt among recruits. "Immediately when Pat announced, we got on the phone," Holly Warlick said. "We were busy." The staff kept the 2012 class intact—a trio of players that will always be loved by Lady Vol fans because they stuck with Tennessee when the program was most vulnerable to having its recruits poached. The high school classes of 2013 and 2014, however, were getting an earful from other colleges and the self-anointed evaluators of girls' basketball. Some of the same coaches who benefited from Summitt's dedication to the game now were using her illness to try to tear down her program. "They used it against us," Warlick said. "Recruits heard: 'That program is history. Pat Summitt isn't there. Warlick is not going to be named coach.' It was brutal."

Davis was subjected to quite a bit of interference and de-committed from Tennessee three months later in early 2012. Davis ended up at Georgia Tech, leaving after two seasons for South Carolina. DeShields, who acknowledged that Summitt's illness affected her decision, chose North Carolina—and had considerable success as a freshman—but had regrets fairly soon after enrolling. She led the Tar Heels to within one game of the Final Four, earned national freshman of the year honors, and announced her intent to transfer at season's end. DeShields followed her heart and chose Tennessee the second time.

The Lady Vols staff and players embarked on the 2011–12 season amid this recruiting environment. They knew every step would be scrutinized. They also knew one other thing: there was no road map for how to proceed. "Here is our scenario: What do we have to do to deal with this and move forward and how do we function and operate?" Lockwood said. "At the same time the highest priority was take care of Pat. Take care of Pat who has taken care of this program and taken care of us for so long. It's time for us to step up even more and take care of her."

7

SEC MEDIA DAY

S EC Media Day always falls in October and features radio, television, print, and online media interview times with all of the men's and women's head basketball coaches and a player representative from each school. The daylong media event begins early in the morning with a break for lunch and a full afternoon of sessions. The coaches and players rotate for individual sit-down interviews with Sirius/XM radio, Fox Sports South, CSS, SEC Digital, and ESPN. It is a busy event under any circumstances, and it is especially so when Pat Summitt is scheduled to arrive two months after announcing she has early onset dementia.

Summitt's video announcement of her diagnosis and September interview with Robin Roberts—the episode aired later in the fall—had been the only national media access to Summitt to date. She had done several interviews with Knoxville media, and the local focus already had shifted to basketball. That wasn't going to be the case in Hoover, Alabama, at SEC Media Day. It was the first chance for dozens of sportswriters and broadcasters

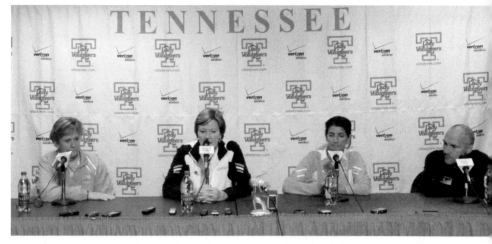

The coaching staff, from left, Holly Warlick, Pat Summitt, Mickie DeMoss, and Dean Lockwood, meet with the media in Knoxville before the 2011–12 season, an appearance typically handled by just the head coach. It was one of the first signs that an unusual season was about to unfold.

to talk to Summitt, and they showed up in droves at the chic Wynfrey Hotel on October 27, 2011.

Print and online sportswriters and local TV stations from various home markets that cover SEC basketball share a large meeting room. The coaches and players sit on elevated tables with four to six places usually occupied at any time as teams rotate through the media schedule. The arrangement, unlike formal press conferences, allows reporters to move about the room to speak to the players and coaches, often with chances for interviews in small groups or even one on one.

(That is never the case for the Kentucky men's coach in 2011 or any year. Kentucky basketball media members seem to arrive by the carload. John Calipari's table was surrounded by press, often three and four rows deep. Then, Summitt showed up and made Kentucky's turnout look like a small gathering.)

Tennessee's turn at the table was timed for right after lunch, and reporters had already staked out spots and set up cameras. Summitt enjoyed lunch with Nikki Caldwell (her former player and now the head coach at LSU), longtime media relations chief Debby Jennings, and assistants Holly Warlick and Mickie DeMoss, who came along for support. Warlick also accompanied

Summitt to the press appearances. Summitt had done fine with Knoxville media members, as she was comfortable and familiar with them, especially the regular beat writers. But this event was packed with reporters in an open room, making it sometimes hard to hear, and Warlick was there to assist as needed. If Summitt appeared to stumble at all, the national media would seize that moment.

The expansive banquet room was filled with writers, photographers, television crews, broadcasters, radio personalities, SEC personnel, coaches, and players. During lunch, Summitt found a table with open spots in the back of the room and chatted with two members of the Knoxville media who were already at the table. A lot of eyes followed Summitt to the table and some well-wishers, especially fellow coaches, stopped by to say hello, but in a delightful peculiarity of Southern manners, the media stayed away and let Summitt enjoy her lunch. She was her usual self at the table, funny and engaging. She asked questions about what had taken place already and joked about being next in the media inquisition line.

ESPN and the other national networks had their own rooms for the event, apart from the general media. This provided the networks with exclusive one-on-one interviews with all players and coaches to air during the upcoming season. When the coaches made their way to the general room, the only TV cameras typically present were those of home markets. Knoxville, as always, had sent all three TV stations to Hoover, but ESPN had set up directly in front of Summitt's table. A crowd of media soon gathered as sportswriters and TV stations that usually didn't pay much attention to women's basketball at SEC Media Day fanned across the room.

The media spilled over from Summitt's designated area with some standing on a nearby dais to get photos. Boom mics were held above her head, cameras clicked and beeped, and longtime SEC observers said it was the largest crowd they had ever seen around one coach. Writers had to fill in behind Summitt and Warlick so they could hear. Male and female coaches and players at the other tables, who were getting little to no attention at this point, sat back and watched. A normally busy room fell mostly quiet on the perimeter as the media descended on one dais set up in front of the center wall. Summitt was the first to enter the room after the lunch break, and the crowd got even deeper as more press members realized she was present and scurried back to work.

ESPN apparently believed Summitt was going to retire and designate Warlick as the head coach. Perhaps Warlick's arrival with Summitt had sparked the rumor. But it didn't seem plausible, and Summitt would never make such an announcement at Media Day in Alabama. News of that level of importance would be handled in Knoxville by the university, not at a conference event two weeks before the season started.

Summitt handled it, as always, with humor, saying a few minutes into her remarks that despite what had been said, she wasn't stepping aside. "I can't wait to get on the court. I am not ready to retire," Summitt said. "Somebody kind of threw that out there today. I may be old as dirt, but I am still trying to win ball games." Warlick interjected at times and said, to much laughter from Summitt and the media, "I am sorry. I am not trying to butt you out Coach Summitt."

"You better not," Summitt said to more laughter.

"I wouldn't dare try," Warlick said.

Summitt handled the 30-minute session well as questions came one after another, most centering on her diagnosis. She answered directly, often eliciting smiles and laughter as she engaged with the media. She addressed her medical condition and handled detailed questions about the team and the upcoming season. She was asked about her favorite things to cook and mentioned grilling food, especially steak, and jalapeno corn. When asked if recruits got to pick a meal, Summitt wittily responded, "It depends on how good they are." She noted how her son Tyler, a Tennessee student and walk-on for the Vols, had become a student of the game and already had suggestions for his mother's team. Finally, the coach was asked whether or not she would remember the referees. Summitt flashed a wicked smile. "I know those referees by name," she said. "I can't forget them."

The Media Day interaction was vintage Summitt as she engaged the media and told jokes. Warlick interjected at times when asked or to add a thought, but Summitt fielded all the questions. "What I want everybody to know is I am doing great," Summitt said. "Every day I want to get up and I want to go to work. That keeps me going." Warlick was attending her first media day—she returned in 2012 as the head coach—and was impressed with the turnout. "I think it's a great tribute to Pat and what she's meant to this program. It's incredible and I was excited for Pat. If anybody deserves it, she does."

Some writers eventually peeled off from the pack and found Vicki Baugh, whose table was set up in the back of the room, giving her a direct view of the crowd around her head coach. Baugh spoke quietly so as to not disrupt the proceedings at Summitt's table. She answered questions about the first practice, season expectations and, of course, Summitt's health. She sat back and watched her surroundings, a visible reminder of Summitt's impact.

The other SEC coaches were peppered with questions about Summitt's diagnosis and her decision to stay on the sideline. Mississippi State Coach Sharon Fanning-Otis, who was a former graduate assistant at Tennessee, likely spoke for the Lady Vols when she issued a friendly challenge to the media to focus on the court now instead of Summitt's medical file. "She made this decision," Fanning-Otis said. "Let her coach. We don't want it to be a memorial for something that hasn't happened. When the ball is tossed, let's play the game."

8

KNOXVILLE MEDIA DAY

The annual Media Day in Knoxville, scheduled on Halloween in 2011, came on the eve of the exhibition opener against Carson-Newman, a small school located in nearby Jefferson County. The game and the statistics don't count, as exhibitions serve as warm-up games. The NCAA requires matchups against college teams as opposed to travel teams of former college players, which had been the case in the past, and if a school opts to schedule a Division I program, the exhibition must be closed to the media and public.

Thus, programs like Tennessee usually schedule Division II or III schools so fans can attend. It gives Tennessee a chance for live competition before the season begins in the arena setting, which is particularly beneficial for freshmen. The benefit for Carson-Newman, which lost in lopsided fashion, was the payment made by Tennessee for the game—vital annual funding for Carson-Newman's athletics department.

Media Day in Knoxville was a much calmer event than the one in Alabama a few days earlier. Summitt was joined at the press conference by all three assistant coaches, and then the arena court was open for one-on-one interviews with all players and coaches, along with an opportunity for the media to watch practice. During this particular practice, the players didn't touch the ball—unless they stole it—minus a few free throws. They had held a scrimmage the previous Saturday, and the defensive performance had been particularly poor. Film study Sunday by the coaches underscored just how subpar it had been, and Summitt was livid. "That is as mad as I've seen her all year," Mickie DeMoss said.

"It was pretty glaring, so we decided to make it strictly a defensive practice. We didn't even want them to touch the ball on offense," Holly Warlick said. This was a session tailor-made for Summitt, who has preached defense for nearly four decades. "What's her whole thing?" Lockwood asked. "That fired her up. I saw her eyes light up about seven minutes into practice, and she was so fired up seeing that. For somebody that loves horses that's like telling them you're going to take them to Churchill Downs for the day." Summitt delivered the thunder at that practice, pointing out slippage in defensive slides, ball denial, and box-outs on the boards. It was an intense practice considering a game was scheduled for the next evening, but the coaches wanted to set the tone for the season.

"It's not that she had so much power over us, but she had a power within her that forced us to continue to push," Meighan Simmons said. "She was still going to push you. I think that created that extra fire in Glory to work even harder and be more dedicated her senior year because Pat had always forced her to become a great player." It was proof that Summitt could still deeply engage her team—and the players responded. They needed her voice, even as they knew things would never be the same.

As expected, the Lady Vols crushed Carson-Newman 105–40. An exhibition game usually draws a few photographers, but both ends of the court were packed in the spots where photographers sit during games, an indication that Summitt on the sideline was going to be a season-long storyline. The announced crowd in terms of ticket sales was 11,500, and while that was a stretch, there were noticeably more fans than in years past at exhibition games. Besides acquiring game film for player teaching purposes, the Tennessee coaches also had their first live run on the sideline since Summitt's diagnosis. Summitt had said she would delegate things to her staff, and that plan had been put into place.

The Lady Eagles wore "We Back Pat" shirts during warmups after a graduate assistant made a quick shopping trip to a local drugstore. Summitt visited with the Carson-Newman players after the game in the locker room, and then Carson-Newman Coach Mike Mincey expressed his appreciation at the post-game press conference. "All the girls are fans. We're all fans of Tennessee. We're all fans of Coach Summitt. She actually came back and signed every one of our shirts. I know she is very busy and a lot of people want things from her, but I think it was very nice of her. All of these girls got to get a picture with her."

Tennessee had one more exhibition game: a 93–45 win November 8 over Union University, a NAIA powerhouse that was overmatched by the length and athleticism of the Lady Vols. After that, it was time for the games to count.

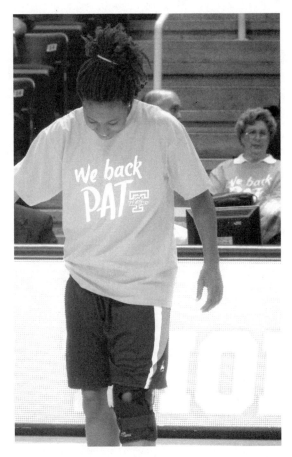

"We Back Pat" shirts became a staple of the opposing team in the final season. Carson-Newman players wore them for the exhibition game.

9

THE 2011–12 SEASON BEGINS

The Lady Vols opened the 2011–12 season at home against Pepperdine.

Pat Summitt standing on the sideline? Check.

Lady Vol fans sitting in Thompson-Boling Arena? Check.

Media packing press row? Check.

Former Tennessee players present for the game? Check, including Lady Vol royalty Chamique Holdsclaw, who was sitting courtside, and Kara Lawson, who was on media row.

A win? Check. The Lady Vols recorded an 89–57 victory over the visiting Waves, who were in Knoxville for a game set up over a year ago because Pepperdine had a player from the South. That player was no longer with the team, but Coach Julie Rousseau welcomed the chance to play in Knoxville. In the Waves' game notes, they referred to it as going to the "basketball mecca" for women's hoops. "Obviously, to coach against Coach Summitt is just a delight and honor," Rousseau said.

Summitt was her same demanding self, even after a 32-point win. "As a coaching staff, we expected a little bit more out of our team in this game," Summitt said. "For a veteran team, I thought we had some opening game jitters. We didn't start strong and kind of faded off and just didn't do what we needed to do. Then, we got it together a little bit." So what was different? It was the first official game led by a head coach who revealed less than three months earlier a diagnosis of early onset dementia.

Before the game, Summitt was honored with the 2011 Mildred "Babe" Didrikson Zaharias Courage Award to thunderous applause from the 12,147 fans in attendance. The award, created by the US Sports Academy, honors an individual who demonstrates courage in overcoming adversity. It would be the first of many awards Summitt would receive as the season progressed, from Sportswoman of the Year by *Sports Illustrated* to the Presidential Medal of Freedom, and one accolade became a source of amusement and an example of Summitt's outlook on her life.

The staff had gathered in a conference room in the basketball office to learn about Summitt's next award. The presentation, while sincere, was effusive, and Summitt felt like it was more a eulogy than a commemoration. "Someone was talking about her and it was something they were going to do for her. It was an honor of some sort. It was always something," Lockwood said. "It was almost like someone was memorializing her: 'Pat, you've done so much. We appreciate you.' She looked at us with that twinkle in her eye and said, 'Well, hell, I'm not dead! I'm still here!' She was very comfortable with our coaching staff. Very honest, very open. There was a comfort level with us."

Summitt was more guarded on the sideline, well aware that the cameras were aimed her way analyzing every move. The game was televised by Sport-South and available on the WatchESPN app. What Summitt decided to do was unprecedented and suddenly she was the national face of Alzheimer's disease. Meanwhile, the coaching staff had the task of keeping matters as normal as possible for the players while crafting a plan for how to run the sideline and timeouts. Coaches attend all sorts of off-season seminars about motivation, strategy, and leadership, but there is no seminar for running a program with a head coach not only battling a serious disease, but also being willing to go public and remain on the sideline. "You are blazing a new trail," Lockwood said.

A critical aspect of coaching basketball is communication with the players, during both timeouts and live action. Of course, some of that communication is directed at officials, and rules of decorum dictate that only one coach is allowed to stand at any given time. The intent is to cut down on verbal harassment of those in stripes. Some egregious conduct has occurred at times when other staff members on the bench in college basketball have targeted officials with verbal outbursts. Lockwood, who is sympathetic to officials and often serves as one during inter-squad scrimmages, doesn't like this rule.

"The minute you stand up, they tell you, 'Sit down. I need you to sit down.' Sometimes I get a little agitated with that because there are times you just can't be heard," he said. "Maybe it's a defensive assignment or you want somebody to change how they're playing somebody. You're going to stand up for a moment, and I totally ignore it. That's basketball." Lockwood would get to his feet, shout some instructions and take a seat on the bench. But the head coach often stands for much of the game, and in 2011–12, Tennessee at times had two of them. Warlick, the associate head coach, was calling the offenses and defenses and shouting at officials. But Summitt also had things to say, especially to the officials, so she would rise, too. Technically, Tennessee could have been issued a technical foul.

"They gave grace to that," Lockwood said. "There could be somebody drop-kicking somebody on the court, but they're going to tell an assistant coach to sit down. But I give them a lot of credit during that time. Nothing was ever said in terms of having two people up. There was grace given to that, and that is as it should have been." During games, the officials would glance at the bench, see both Summitt and Warlick on their feet, and swallow the whistles. "We were both up," Warlick said. "That was out of respect for Pat. I think it was an understood rule that they were going to let both of us get up." Warlick was up most of the time, but if Summitt saw something she didn't like, she would leap off the bench—and it invigorated the crowd every time. Meighan Simmons smiled about the arrangement: "If it came to a ref and a bad call, it was Pat," she said.

It was beneficial to the players, especially as Summitt yielded the huddle to her assistants, knowing she could not keep up as clearly with the second-by-second action. The players needed Summitt's presence, even as they battled emotionally every day with the realization that their head coach would never be the same. "I hold my emotions in, but those emotions I wore on my sleeve a little bit," Simmons said. "During the games if Holly was talking in the huddle and drawing up a play, I would be looking up at Pat like, 'Are you going to say something? Did you say something?' I think it wore on me because of who she was to me and how she motivated me."

The players accept the fishbowl that their lives become as recognizable athletes; the tradeoff is being able to take the court and get lost in the game they love. This season meant some of those tradeoff moments would be stolen, as their eyes darted in huddles and they watched Summitt adjust to her new reality as a head coach. "It was extremely difficult," Taber Spani said. "One of the hardest parts was seeing her internal struggle. You just knew how frustrated she was. And yet how selfless she was and how she wanted to be there for us. You just felt for her so much. All she wanted to do was focus on her team and coaching and doing what she had done for the past 37 years. And all of a sudden she couldn't do what she wanted to do in the capacity that she had before."

Amid this sea change, a team desperately wanted to get their coach to a Final Four. They knew the clock was ticking on Summitt's career.

10

MANIFESTATION OF DEMENTIA

Pat Summitt made a Tip-off Club appearance in January 2012 that showed how engaged she still was with her program. But dementia is a disease that produces good days and bad ones, and that certainly was the case with Summitt. With the benefit of hindsight, those close to Summitt now have a better understanding of how the disease both hides and progresses. "None of us knew," Glory Johnson said. "The little forgetful things that she was doing, we thought it was normal. Everyone forgets once in a while. And when she told us we were like, 'Man, all those incidents before? We should have seen it.' But we didn't. So, it was really, really tough.'"

Johnson recalls the Sweet 16 matchup against Baylor in Memphis, a 77–62 loss on March 27, 2010. The Lady Vols trailed by just two points at halftime, 30–28, but Baylor's Brittney Griner erupted in the second half while Johnson was planted on the bench. She was the Lady Vols' most physical player, though Kelley Cain had secured the win over Baylor earlier that season in Knoxville with her defense against Griner. Johnson didn't enter the second half until just less than six minutes remained with the Lady Vols trailing by

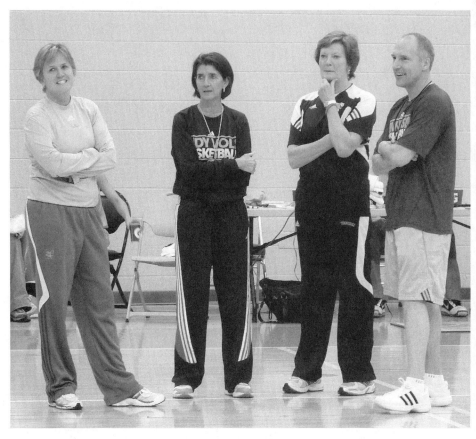

Holly Warlick, Mickie DeMoss, Pat Summitt, and Dean Lockwood, during a final season practice.

five. She exited two minutes later with the deficit at six points. When Johnson reentered with one minute remaining, the Lady Vols were down 12.

"I remember the Baylor coach looking at me, waiting for Pat to put me in," Johnson said. "At the end of the game, Pat told me, 'I don't know what I was thinking. I feel like I should have put you in well before.' She was standing there with her arms crossed, and she was quiet. That is not her. I talked to her afterwards and said, 'We'll get them next time.' That was one of the moments for me that indicated something was wrong."

Summitt had been annoyed that season with Johnson, as her effort could be sporadic. She knew Johnson had barely tapped her potential, and Summitt was often tougher on players she thought were underachieving. "Pat wasn't quite herself in that game," said Lockwood, though he noted the game plan had been to get Angie Bjorklund and Shekinna Stricklen open with ball screens on the perimeter. Post players Cain and Alyssia Brewer were adept at setting screens, so they were often on the court. Bjorklund and Stricklen could drain three-pointers, and the plan worked: they got great looks, but they misfired too often.

Mickie DeMoss was hired as an assistant coach two months later in May 2010 after years of being away from the program. She noticed her longtime friend wasn't the same. "She was still involved, but she wasn't running practice like she used to, running team meetings like she used to. She deferred a lot of that to Holly and Dean," DeMoss said.

The media had noticed some changes, too. Summitt had long been able to multitask to the extreme, and her ability to process and retain information with pinpoint focus—no matter how fast it was being fired at her—was legendary. She could accomplish in half a day what would take a week for someone else. Summitt was the CEO of Lady Vols basketball, so if there was any slippage, it was going to be noted. But her rheumatoid arthritis would flare, and the medications for that condition can cause some confusion. It was easy to dismiss the symptoms as side effects from the medicine, especially since there were plenty of times Summitt seemed the same.

Jenny Moshak, who was called JMo by the players, had been by Summitt's side for 26 years, including her time as a graduate assistant. During the 2010–11 season, which would become the penultimate one for Summitt, Moshak saw changes. "I noticed a couple of things. There was one particular time directly related to me. I called her each day with basically an injury report. I called her that morning and told her of a player not being able to practice. She came into the gym and kind of came firmly up to me and said, 'Why isn't she practicing?' And I said, 'Pat, we talked about that this morning.' She said, 'Oh, OK. Well, tell me again.' Then, she was fine with it. It was so unlike Pat. Unbelievably unlike Pat. She could have 16 things on her plate, and she would remember them."

"A couple of other times in huddle with a lot of information coming in and it not being processed the way she was used to processing it . . . again this is hindsight," Moshak continued. "And now it makes sense. I noticed some mood swings. She would get frustrated and angrier more quickly. Looking back, that was probably being frustrated. She was mad at herself and the situation."

Vicki Baugh also noticed a change during that 2010–11 season. She was in her fourth year on campus and had been a part of the 2008 team when

Summitt was in her prime as a motivator and strategist. Still, the diagnosis was unexpected. "I was surprised when I found out, but I knew something was wrong just from when I would talk to Pat," Baugh said. "There was a lot of time I didn't practice so I would be on the sideline, and I would talk to Pat. She would always come check on me on the sidelines. There was something that was a little off. I would ask JMo, 'Is Pat alright?' I knew something was a little off that year, but I had no idea what it was."

Taber Spani was a sophomore that season—she would be a junior in Summitt's final year—and she also detected something was awry. "Looking back, I can see little things, maybe including the coaches more and removing herself a tad, though she was absolutely still the head coach," Spani said. "I wasn't completely thrown off guard, but you can't ever prepare for an announcement like that. There's no way. I did know something wasn't right."

11

ANGIE BJORKLUND

Angie Bjorklund sat upright, surrounded by cameras and sportswriters asking her about her final game as a Lady Vol, a 73–59 loss to Notre Dame in the Elite Eight in Dayton, Ohio, on March 28, 2011. The locker room at Dayton Arena was small, and the coaches sat on chairs just a few feet from the players, the sounds of the Fighting Irish celebration ringing through the walls. Locker rooms often have separate areas for coaches and players to meet before gathering in a common area, but this one could barely fit a team. Four years ago, this same room was the scene of jubilation as the Lady Vols were headed to the Final Four in Cleveland. In 2011, it was somber. The stale air felt like a smothering blanket. A team that the day before was confident it could reach a Final Four had a desultory showing on defense and an anemic performance on offense.

Author's note: Angie Bjorklund was present for Pat Summitt at the peak of her game and for the gradual decline. Her story is an important one.

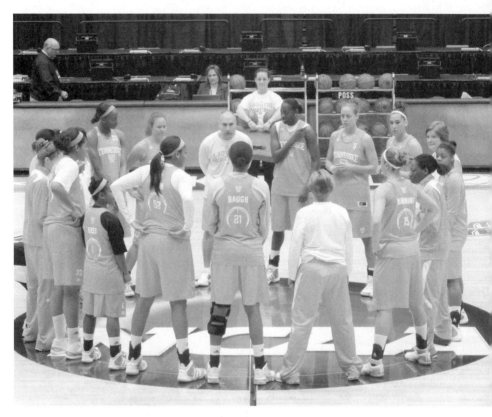

The team gathers at a practice in the Dayton Regional in Ohio in March 2011. Five months later, Pat Summitt's diagnosis would be made public. It was in Dayton that the change in Summitt's demeanor on the bench and with the media became noticeably different.

Bjorklund was shattered. She had wanted to lead her team back to the Final Four as a senior. Her eyes were red, but the program's all-time leading three-point shooter handled each question with poise and grace. A small space was made even more cramped by the presence of media members trying to interview players, and when those carrying TV cameras shifted, they had to be careful not to sideswipe anyone with their equipment. Inside this cauldron sat Summitt within earshot of everyone, seething over the loss.

I write for *InsideTennessee*, a website that covers the Vols and Lady Vols, and asked Summitt to discuss the reasons for the defeat. Her eyes narrowed, and she unloaded in a response full of anger and frustration. It wasn't characteristic of Summitt, who would outline losses in stark terms

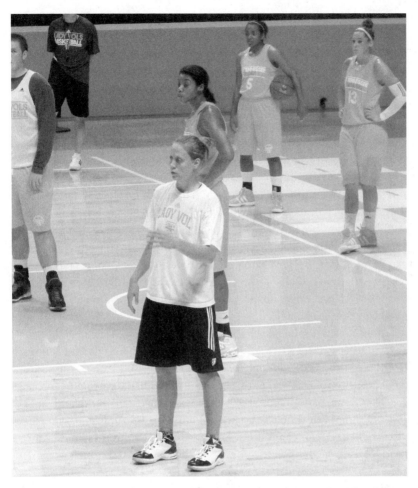

Angie Bjorklund returned to campus on occasion to practice with the team during the 2011–12 season. Pat Summitt's diagnosis brought some clarity to Bjorklund about how her senior season unfolded in 2010–11. Vicki Baugh, Ariel Massengale, and Taber Spani are behind her.

but without vitriol. Those sitting nearby glanced at Summitt, somewhat taken aback. Two months later, a trip to the Mayo Clinic would reveal her condition. "I firmly believe she was frustrated; she knew something wasn't sharp so she was getting upset," Jenny Moshak said.

Even after the worst postseason defeat in Tennessee history (the loss to Ball State in the first round of the 2009 NCAA Tournament), Summitt, while peeved to say the least, had answered media questions at length, offering both insightful and straightforward remarks. Bjorklund, just a sophomore that season on a team with seven freshmen, had been the one who delivered a declaration that players needed to either get to work or exit. But now it was 2011, and Bjorklund was about to remove her Lady Vol jersey for the last time. And when Summitt was asked to talk about the senior right after the coach's takedown of the team, Summitt's face noticeably softened, and she said she would miss her senior and all that Bjorklund had done for Tennessee.

Bjorklund was the 10th rookie to start her first game as a Lady Vol and had quite the start to her career in orange and white with a championship as a freshman. The somewhat absent-minded Bjorklund had her national title ring sitting on a dresser in her off-campus apartment the following season until her father saw it while visiting and suggested a safety deposit box in her hometown of Spokane, Washington, might be a better location. "I was like, 'Ang, this is pretty valuable,'" Jim Bjorklund said. "She said, 'This is really cool. I don't think I'd ever wear it because it's really gaudy and heavy and showy.' I said, 'How about if I just take it home for you and put it in a safe place?' She said, 'OK.'"

After Alexis Hornbuckle hit the shot to put Tennessee ahead in the semi-final game against LSU in the Final Four in 2008, Bjorklund chest-bumped Hornbuckle and then suddenly remembered to get back on defense. After the game, Summitt reminded the players to act like they had been there before—Tennessee was the defending champion—and Bjorklund smiled and reminded her coach that she had not. Her titles also include three SEC regular season championships and three SEC Tournament crowns. Bjorklund made the honor roll every semester at Tennessee and earned 2010 SEC Scholar-Athlete of the Year honors.

Her fixation on Tennessee had started in middle school. She read Summitt's books—the inspirational business one, *Reach for the Summit*, and *Raise the Roof*, an account of the undefeated 1997–98 season, both written by Sally Jenkins, a best-selling author and sportswriter for the Washington Post. Bjorklund also watched the HBO documentary on the 10-loss "Cinderella Season" in 1997 that ended in a national championship. "That book, *Raise the Roof*, she read that twice," mother Kris Bjorklund said. "They're reading the English book in class, and she has the book and then has Pat's book behind it reading it. She wanted to play for Pat Summitt. That was her dream."

Summitt smiled when she was told of Bjorklund tucking one of the coach's books into a textbook at school. "It's very fitting for Angie because sometimes she's not always focused on what she needs to be focused on," Summitt said. That's a quintessential Summitt quotation—an underlying challenge to a player mixed with humor. But Summitt was thrilled that Bjorklund chose to cross the country to play at Tennessee. She is Summitt's kind of player. "She's a gym rat. I love gym rats. Love 'em."

"When I was little, I'm talking middle school, I was carrying my basketball everywhere," Angie Bjorklund said. "I'd be in the mall bouncing my ball. People would be like, 'Who's the kid?'"

Jami Bjorklund (now Jami Schaefer after marrying Drew Schaefer), Angie's older sister by two years, also played basketball, and the sisters squared off against each other. "We played one-on-one for hours," Schaefer said. "She tried to beat me but she couldn't because I was bigger than her. In high school Angie would go to the gym and play pickup with the guys all the time. She'd ride her bike with her basketball. She was always in the gym."

Bjorklund attended Summitt's basketball camp while in high school and wanted to commit on the spot. She called Jim Bjorklund, who advised his youngest daughter to come home, think about it away from the excitement of being in Knoxville, and then make the decision: "I remember when she was at camp. She called home a couple of times and said, 'Dad, I'm on Summitt Boulevard, you can't believe this.' And then she goes, 'Dad, I've got to go. There's a black Mercedes pulling up and it's Coach Summitt. I've got to go!' She hangs the phone up. She calls back the next day and said Coach basically offered her a scholarship. She goes, 'Dad, what do I do?' She really wanted to take it right then. I said, 'You've got to calm down and say I'm very flattered and will probably take it, but I'm going to think about it for a while.'"

Bjorklund returned home, checked other schools, thought it over and committed to Tennessee while a junior in high school. Her commitment never wavered, and she arrived in Knoxville a few weeks after turning 18 years old. "I came in at such a perfect time," Bjorklund said. "I got to play with some of the best players that ever came through the Tennessee program. I got to be coached by Pat and be a part of her last championship. Just saying it is amazing. You don't think about it until everything's done, after you leave and look back. Wow. I was part of something really special."

The Lady Vols had long been aware of Bjorklund, and an assist for Tennessee's early interest should be credited to Fred Crowell, the leader of Northwest Basketball Camps. His camps are Christian-based and he travels the country and overseas with players from youngsters to post-college. "I have to give a lot of credit to Fred Crowell," Pat Summitt said. "He knew Angie, and I had worked with his guys at Baden's (basketball manufacturer) clinics. He told me about Angie. She was in the seventh or eighth grade when he first mentioned it. She had gone to his camps quite a bit. He said, 'Pat, I've never told you about anyone, but I'm telling you about this kid, and she's really, really good.' He was the first one to tell me about her."

When Summitt overheard Stanford Coach Tara VanDerveer talking about Bjorklund in 2004 at a summer basketball event, she stepped up her efforts. Summitt left the room to call her secretary, Katie Wynn, to get Crowell's contact info. She then placed a call to Crowell. "I called to find out where she was going to be. She was going to be in Arizona for an AAU competition. I called Dean and I said, 'Get on the plane and go to Arizona.'"

Dean Lockwood was in Kentucky when he took the call from Summitt. It was July 28, 2004—Lockwood keeps meticulous travel records—and he was ready for a new location. "I was in Louisville at a camp at Bellarmine College, and for us, at that point, there weren't a lot of players there so I was very happy to leave," Lockwood said. "I called our travel agent and by 4 or 4:30 I was on a plane. It was the summer of 2004—I was just on board (as a new assistant coach at Tennessee). Angie was going into her sophomore year."

Lockwood landed in Tempe and still remembers his initial assessment of Bjorklund. "A skilled kid, especially to be so young. I am somebody who is more conservative than I am superlative when it comes to players. As enthusiastic as I am (on the practice court and during games), when it comes to evaluating I might see somebody and say, 'Oh yeah, she's solid.' But I thought this kid is very skilled. For as young as she is to be as skilled as she is, that's what impressed me."

Angie's sister Jami played basketball for Gonzaga, her hometown school, and the Bulldogs were a finalist for Angie because of those sister connections. But Angie's heart was set on orange and white. The city sent her away with its blessing, as did Kelly Graves, the coach of Gonzaga. "Oh my goodness, how can you pass up on Tennessee?" Graves said. "You grow up as a kid and that's where you want to go and you have the opportunity to go there and play for arguably the best coach in our business, not just the women's side, in basketball in a storied program like that? You want her to go. That's where she belongs."

Spokane is well known for its love of basketball, and the Gonzaga arena was packed when Tennessee came to town in late December 2008 for Bjorklund's home game during one of the worst snowstorms in the city's history. Snow piles in the parking lot exceeded 10 feet. Cars parked on the street were buried in snow.

When Bjorklund was introduced before the Tennessee-Gonzaga game on December 30, the crowd roared so loud her name was drowned out on the public address system. Every time Bjorklund hit a shot, the crowd cheered. "I think that was mainly the Bjorklunds, the whole cheering section," Bjorklund said. The extended Bjorklund clan and friends filled a section and wore special gray T-shirts that commemorated the game (her parents wore "TennZaga" T-shirts to support both daughters), but fans wearing just Gonzaga gear also openly cheered for Bjorklund.

After the game and media interviews, Bjorklund returned to the court and expected a few family members to be waiting for her. Instead, a crowd of Gonzaga fans young and old surrounded her in the stands to get autographs. She stayed for nearly 30 minutes to accommodate each request before her family returned her to the team hotel (Tennessee wasn't departing Spokane until the next morning), and her coach also drew quite a crowd. "When I came out I was just expecting my family to be there," said Bjorklund, who has athletic basketball genes. Her uncle, Steve Ranniger, played at Oregon. Her maternal grandfather, Duane Ranniger, played at Washington State. Her paternal grandfather, Leon Bjorklund, ran track at Washington.

The team departed the state of Washington the next morning for a cross-country journey to New Jersey and a matchup with Rutgers. Tennessee was trailing at the half in that game, 33–13, and CBS's in-locker room camera aired Summitt challenging Bjorklund about putting on a show in Spokane and being a no-show in Piscataway. Bjorklund didn't react on camera except to nod in agreement, and Summitt's tone wasn't derisive. It was simply matter of fact. "That's how Coach is," Bjorklund said. "She was getting into me the whole first half a little more aggressively than that. I think they filmed the not-so-crazy part at halftime. That's her coaching style—sort of short and to the point and staring at you. That's why she's the best." Bjorklund ended up with 12 points against Rutgers, and Tennessee staged the biggest comeback in school history with the 55–51 win.

The Chicago Sky drafted Bjorklund in April 2011 after her senior season ended, but a lingering right foot injury led to her release in late July. She had injured the foot midway through her senior year at Tennessee and missed some games and practice before returning to the starting lineup in the postseason. Bjorklund returned to Knoxville to undergo rehab with Jenny Moshak. It was very common for former Lady Vols to seek Moshak for help with their comebacks long after they had left Tennessee. The players trusted her implicitly to get them back on the court. Candace Parker had torn her ACL in high school and dealt with a different and serious injury on the same knee that wasn't diagnosed until she got to Tennessee. She credits Moshak with saving her career.

Bjorklund had barely been out of college when Summitt went public with her diagnosis. She returned to Tenenssee a few months later to rehab a foot injury with Jenny Moshak. "I remember just sitting down to talk to Pat and it's not an easy thing. At one point we were both in tears. We're part of her family. That is what she would always say and that's how I feel."

Bjorklund has the perspective of playing for Summitt at her absolute best and then being present for the subtle changes that occurred over time. "From my freshman year to my senior year I would say that the biggest change that I saw was the changing of the roles of the coaching staff. My freshman year she was more running the show in terms of calling plays, calling defenses. It was hard to tell because at Tennessee it is so unique because everyone plays a big role on that staff. Pat has always made the final call, but she has always had such great support from her staff. But slowly with time you saw it. Pat started to say less in the huddles, during timeouts. By senior year, Holly and Mickie started stepping up a little bit in those moments."

However, nothing Bjorklund witnessed ever caused her to believe Summitt had a serious illness. "No, no. It didn't even go through my head because she was still the same Pat. Her intensity on the court, her genuine personality off the court, that didn't change. Her presence was always there. She was the same intense Pat that got on the players, held us accountable. You couldn't take a day off with her no matter what. She walks in and her presence just brings this intensity. It was such a subtle and slow change from my freshman to senior year that you really didn't see it until after she came out and said, 'I have dementia.'"

Bjorklund, who played professionally in Israel and France, became the director of basketball operations at Santa Clara and then took a position with the women's basketball program at Idaho. Aspiring to be a head coach, Bjorklund savors her memories of time with Summitt: "That's when I've always had the most genuine times with coach is when you meet with her one on one. A player can be honest with her, and she was honest with me. We had a freaked-out moment and hugged and cried. I thanked her for everything. It was a good moment to get back with her, not only about her illness, but also her. I told her how much she's been a great part of my life and how she's positively impacted it. It was a good moment. I sure miss her. That's for sure."

12

CANDACE PARKER

When Candace Parker arrived in Knoxville in August 2004, the Lady Vols had last won a national title in 1998. By Tennessee's standards, it was a serious drought, and Parker was expected to return the Lady Vols to the proverbial promised land.

She did, leaving town with two national championship rings in 2007 and 2008, but her Tennessee debut was delayed by major knee surgery as a freshman, causing Parker to sit out the 2004–05 season. During the 2005–06 season, the starting point guard transferred midseason, and Alexis Hornbuckle slid from the wing to take over the position. But late in the season trying to save a loose ball, she landed hard on the baseline and broke her wrist. Hornbuckle returned for the NCAA Tournament but had to wear

---

Author's note: Candace Parker restored Tennessee to prominence on a national stage. Hers is a story of the quintessential Pat Summitt on and off the court.

a soft, almost club-like cast. Needless to say, it affected her shooting and ball handling, and the Lady Vols lost in the Elite Eight in Cleveland, Ohio, to North Carolina in 2006. Of course, that also was the site of great triumph one year later.

By the 2007–08 season, Parker, who had attended multiple summer school sessions, had nearly graduated. She had just one class in her final semester, and it met in the evening, so Parker had plenty of time to work out in the gym and stop by the basketball offices outside of official practices and meetings. She took full advantage and stopped by Summitt's office often to talk, sometimes about basketball but often about life.

While in college, Parker met Shelden Williams, a former Duke stand-out and NBA player. During the national title game in Cleveland in 2007, Williams was in the stands watching Parker lead Tennessee to its first natty (in the basketball vernacular) since 1998. They would later marry and have a daughter, Lailaa, but while in college, they dated and tried to see each other when they could—certainly not easy since Parker was a student and basketball player and Williams was a pro athlete.

Summitt always scheduled a "home" game for her players, and in Parker's case, it was January 2, 2008, against DePaul in Chicago. Classes were out, so the team had arrived two days early so they could enjoy the city. Summitt, a clothes hound, also wanted to go shopping, something she did every time the team played in Chicago, New York, or the San Francisco area. Williams made the trip to Chicago for Parker's homecoming game, so the two enjoyed New Year's Eve together. But Parker didn't make it back to the team hotel by curfew, and Summitt was calling both of them to determine why her All-American forward wasn't in her room. Parker saw multiple missed calls from Summitt on her phone at the same time Williams' phone rang. Parker heard her future husband say, "Yes ma'am," several times. Parker knew she was in trouble.

The evening game had long been sold out, and Parker's family members sat behind the bench wearing T-shirts with her No. 3 on the back and her photo on the front. Summitt, who treated her all-star players the same as her walk-ons, benched Parker for the first half. "I apologized to my team-mates, my coaches, my family and friends, and Chicago in general for not being able to play in the first half," Parker said. Parker did more than that: autograph seekers always approach the Lady Vol players and coaches as they walk to the team bus on the road, and a huge crowd had gathered hoping to get Parker's signature. It was bitter cold and approaching midnight, but

Parker, after first getting permission, stayed behind to sign every autograph. Her mother, Sara Parker, took her to the team hotel.

Parker readily accepted Summitt's decision. The two had become very close—and remained so—and Parker knew Summitt did what a head coach must to maintain a team's respect. "What's so special about Coach is that a lot of people can be great coaches. They know Xs and Os and stuff like that. But she genuinely cares," Parker said. "That is who she is." Summitt puts her players first. No matter what, if a player called, she answered the phone. Summitt's phone could buzz 10 times in a 30-minute interview. She would glance and ignore, never even pausing, unless the incoming call indicated it was a current or former player. Then, the interview was put on hold until Summitt answered the call and determined whether the matter needed to be addressed right then or could wait a few minutes.

Parker stopped by Summitt's office often, and the coach always made time for her. A conversation that was intended to take 15 minutes or so could last two hours. "I would open the door and go in there and start off talking basketball and two hours later we're talking about politics and what I want to do when I graduate, whether Shelden was the one for me, my parents, my fears, my excitement, everything," Parker said. "I remember looking at her with so much awe and thinking those conversations would happen all the time because they did even after I graduated. I look back now and I really treasure and really respect all the things that she taught me."

Lailaa was a surprise. While Candace and Shelden intended to get married and have children, Lailaa arrived ahead of the couple's schedule. The pair eloped to Lake Tahoe, Nevada, and tied the knot in the fall of 2008. Six months later, Lailaa was born on May 13, 2009. Parker's WNBA career was slightly delayed that season, but she returned to the court for the summer league just six weeks after giving birth. The marriage wasn't a surprise. When Parker was still in college, she had gotten a tattoo of a lock on her wrist. The key that fit the lock was tattooed on Shelden's wrist. He also passed the Summitt test. "Sometimes Pat would hug and kiss Shelden before she did me," Parker recalls. "She would give Shelden a big hug."

One of the first phone calls Parker made when she found out she was pregnant was to her former college coach. "I was pregnant with Lailaa and nobody knew. I was calling to tell her," Parker said. "She was like, 'Oh, my goodness. We have another grandchild. We have somebody who is going to sign with Tennessee in 18 years. This is great. I am so excited for you. Candace, this such a blessing.' The next day, I open my door, and it is all this Tennessee stuff on my doorstep that Pat sent. In all aspects of life, she cares, she's there."

Parker saw absolutely no signs of any decline in Summitt during her time at Tennessee. Summitt would occasionally misplace her keys or phone, but that wasn't unusual. Anyone who watched Summitt on the sideline during those championship runs in 2007 and 2008 would have seen the head coach in her finest form, as both a motivator and a strategist. "I forget my keys. I don't know where I placed my purse. She is just busy doing stuff," Parker said. "She was talking on the phone. She was putting on her makeup. She was making sure what time Tyler's teacher-parent conferences were. She was making sure she had time to go home and cook dinner. She would go to Tyler's games. She was recruiting. She was doing a million things."

The indications that something could be wrong began to appear during the 2009–10 and 2010–11 seasons. But Summitt was still functioning at an extremely high level, and a side effect of her arthritis medication—Summitt's career as a basketball player had taken its toll on her joints—was forgetfulness or confusion, so it was easy to pinpoint that as the cause of any hiccups along the way. "At the end of the next year and into the following year was where she started having problems and people started noticing things," Parker said.

Parker plays basketball nearly year-round, as she is able to earn a seven-figure salary in Russia. As a result, she wasn't often stateside. Between a professional career overseas and the WNBA in the summer, Parker kept up with Summitt mostly with fairly frequent telephone calls. Nothing alarmed her during those exchanges. "Every time I would call her, I would hear, 'Caaandace,'" Parker said, imitating Summitt's southern accent. "That is how she answered the phone every time. Even now, I hear that voice."

Parker, who called Summitt on a regular basis and always on Mother's Day, remembers the urgency in the voices of Dean Lockwood and Nikki Caldwell in August 2011 about needing to call Summitt. "I was in Washington, D.C., and we were going to play the Mystics. Nikki Caldwell told me I needed to call Pat. I was like, 'OK, why do people keep telling me I need to talk to her when I talk to her all the time and everything is fine?' When Dean called me, immediately I thought she had cancer. And I already prepared my 'OK, we're going to beat it' speech." When she reached Summitt, Parker heard the word dementia.

"I was taken aback. I told her I am here, I am always going to be here. Of course Pat was, 'I am OK. I am going to be fine. Tyler's got me doing puzzles.' Typical Pat. I just told her I love you, and we're going to fight this. And she just said, 'Yeah, we are, we're going to fight this for sure.'" The news was devastating to Parker, as it was to everyone who heard it, whether a former player or a fan who had admired the iconic coach from afar. It took a while for Parker to find any semblance of peace.

"After some reflection and after talking to Dean, we realized Pat is going to deal with this better than anybody or any of us would. We didn't think it was possible for her to touch more people than she does in women's basketball but now she's going to touch far more people. She is going to have a lasting impact on a lot of people's lives." Sure enough, Summitt started her foundation to heighten awareness of the disease and raise much-needed funds for research. Adam Waller, a student manager for the Lady Vols basketball team from 2001 to 2005, now handles community relations for the foundation. One of the items sold by Summitt's foundation is a rubber orange-and-purple "Fierce Courage" bracelet. It is on Parker's wrist when she takes the court.

"I wear Pat Summitt's bracelet every time I step on the floor, every game, every moment," Parker said. "Lailaa gets really upset because the bracelets don't fit her, and she wants to wear it. I told her when we go see Pat, we will have Adam make her a smaller bracelet. She said, 'Mommy wears the bracelet because Pat Summitt is tough. She's sick, but she's really tough.' That is what she explains to people about why mommy wears the bracelet."

13

COAST TO COAST

Pat Summitt always put together a national schedule, so coast-to-coast trips were common during the season. She wanted women's basketball to reach as many fans as possible, and she was willing to take her team anywhere to promote the game. Summitt was one of the first to say yes to Connecticut and Geno Auriemma when his fledging program needed national exposure, but she ended the series in 2007, in part because she suspected recruiting shenanigans that she didn't expect from an elite coach.

It was Tennessee's turn to renew the contract, and the next game would have been played in Knoxville with the Lady Vols' dominant trio of Candace Parker, Nicky Anosike, and Alexis Hornbuckle in their senior season. Tennessee had won three consecutive matchups against Connecticut and a home game likely meant a fourth. But Summitt had reached her breaking point in what had started as a respectful and competitive series and devolved into one of acrimony and insults.

By 2000, Auriemma was ready to take Summitt's national mantle. UConn had won the national title in 1995, while Tennessee had won three straight in

1996, 1997, and 1998. During the 2000 Final Four in Philadelphia—UConn defeated the Lady Vols for the national title; the Lady Vols lost point guard Ace Clement, a Philly native, to an ankle sprain the morning of the game in shoot-around—Auriemma joked to the media about two legendary cheesesteak operations, one called Geno's, the other Pat's. He said Geno's was new and modern and Pat's was old and outdated. Their difference in age was less than two years.

To an outsider, it looked like classic Auriemma humor, and the Northeast media inhaled his words. After Connecticut won the national title, a *Hartford Courant* columnist wrote: *Geno Auriemma returned to Philly and made a statement as bold and beautiful as the signature John Hancock once hung on the British down the street from here.* It wasn't intended as hyperbole; the outcome of a championship basketball game was being compared to the country's signature document. Auriemma had seduced the Northeast media.

To those who knew the escalating undercurrent of tension between the head coaches, and the fact Summitt had no desire to fade away on the national scene, the remarks about the cheesesteaks joints carried intent and went well beyond humor. Still, Summitt stayed silent and kept playing. She was a tireless promoter of the game and knew the series had energized the sport on the national scene. But seven years later she had finally had enough, with recruiting shenanigans being the final straw.

So in 2007, after defeating Connecticut on its home court—the game in which Parker dunked in front of a national television audience—Summitt was done. She knew that would be the last game against UConn in the regular season, and she held her ground despite continued attempts, especially by ESPN and the Northeast media, to renew the series. Connecticut media, apparently trying to force the issue, reported that Tennessee had declined to sign the contract. That wasn't possible, however, because it was Tennessee's turn to set the parameters of the contract—it flipped every two years—so a contract by Tennessee didn't even exist.

Auriemma called Summitt and unleashed a fusillade of profanity. She held the phone away from her ear and it was so loud that her son Tyler, who was then in high school, came in the room to see what was wrong. Summitt mouthed the word, "Geno," and Tyler rolled his eyes and left the room. Auriemma told Summitt he needed the series. Summitt told Auriemma she considered him a coaching peer and if the recruiting playing field wasn't level between the two of them, she wasn't playing his team in the regular season. When the media later asked Summitt why she ended the series, she said, "Ask Geno; he knows." And he did.

The coast-to-coast travel continued.

In December 2011, the Lady Vols were preparing for a two-game swing to the Northeast for matchups against DePaul in the Maggie Dixon Classic in New York's Madison Square Garden and against Rutgers in Piscataway, New Jersey. On December 5, 2011, a few days before the team departed, Summitt was selected as *Sports Illustrated*'s Sportswoman of the Year for her lifetime achievements. The Lady Vols had just returned to Knoxville after a 73–57 win over Texas in Austin, and final exams were underway that week.

Two things happened at the morning practice: the Lady Vols assembled for a very short session, and the *SI* news was released about Summitt. It wasn't mentioned in the team's pre-practice gathering at center court—Summitt was low key about any honors that came her way—but senior forward Glory Johnson had somehow already heard about it. "We were doing the first drill at practice, Pat was standing right next to me, and Glory came back from a rep and said, 'Congratulations.' And Pat said, 'Thank you,'" Lockwood recalls. The assistant coaches had been given a heads up about the award before it was announced Monday morning, but the players were arriving for practice at the same time that *SI* released the news. "It was practice as usual," Lockwood said. "We came in and watched tape."

Summitt shared the award with Duke Coach Mike Krzyzewski, who became the winningest coach in Division I men's basketball history with his 903rd victory that season. Summitt holds the overall Division I record with 1,098 career wins. The college basketball coaches previously selected for the recognition by *Sports Illustrated* were UCLA's John Wooden and North Carolina's Dean Smith. "That is pretty heady company," Lockwood said. "You think of all the great coaches there who have been in college basketball, oh my gosh, it's like a hallowed hall."

The award gave Summitt another platform to promote her message that dementia didn't define her and she could continue to live her life. However, Summitt has always had a narrow focus, especially when it came to basketball, and her thoughts were with her team, as was apparent that day when she made no mention of the upcoming *SI* cover during the practice session. "Pat by her nature is very humble and gracious," Lockwood said two years before Summitt's death. "She will talk about the great players and things of that nature. It's hard to know what she really (thinks about the honor). I would love, in a quiet moment when she is looking over that back river, to hear what she thinks as she processes this and thinks, 'Wow.' I do think it is kind of affirmation that, 'Hey, you know what? It's been a heck of a run so far. Things are different, but things are still good here.'"

Things were business as usual on the practice court. It was shorter than usual but that was by design with the players in the midst of final exams. "You can always tell when it is exam week," Summitt said. "The players are so focused on finishing up the semester strong. We always take that into account with our practice days and off days this week. This group is very focused academically." With that in mind, the session lasted a little over an hour, including film, so the players could devote more time to studying. The next day would be an off day to allow a full day away from basketball.

With the media's arrival to interview Summitt, the players slowly became aware of the *SI* recognition. "It's fantastic," freshman point guard Ariel Massengale said. "She deserves it . . . everything that she's been through and how strong she is and a role model for all of her fans, people all around the world." Summitt spoke to the assembled media after practice: "I am humbled by it. I just really appreciate this honor. I never, ever thought about anything like this." Summitt was able to spend time during her career with Wooden, Smith, and Krzyzewski and talk hoops. "I have been in their company, and I can just tell you that I am always learning from everybody else," Summitt said. "It's not all about me. It's about the other people that have influenced my life." Accompanied by her son, Tyler, Summitt traveled to Manhattan on December 6, 2011, to receive the award. She spoke live during the presentation to tremendous applause. "I just want to say what an honor it is to be a part of such a great award in the company of so many amazing people that have done so much."

Summitt returned to Knoxville, and two days later, Massengale severely dislocated a finger on her left hand while trying to scoop up a loose ball in practice the day before the team departed for New York. Although Massengale was on the team plane, she was unavailable to play, which was particularly disappointing since she is from the Chicago area and the first opponent on the two-game road swing was DePaul. Massengale missed the next month of the season, and it was a severe blow to Tennessee. She was so skilled that Summitt would publicly declare, when Massengale was a high school senior, that she would start at Tennessee. Summitt's proclamation about Massengale was something she would say privately to people she trusted (and Massengale indeed started as a Lady Vol freshman), but not publicly. Dementia can loosen the brain's filters, and in hindsight, it was one of those remarks that made more sense after Summitt's diagnosis was revealed.

The team arrived on a Friday and held practice Saturday at the New York Athletic Club, a hotel and facility so swanky that there is a dress code for public areas and athletic attire is allowed only in the gym areas. The

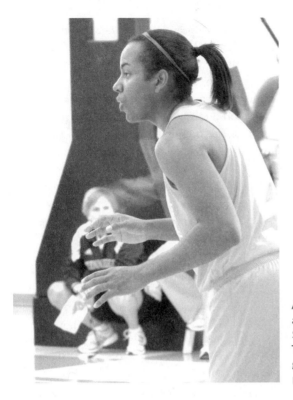

Ariel Massengale was able to play for Pat Summitt for one season. The freshman point guard became a key player in her first season.

staff there had always treated Summitt well and were somehow even more gracious on this trip. "The practice facility is in the hotel, so that's really convenient," Glory Johnson said. Freshman Isabelle Harrison was also well aware of the significance of Madison Square Garden, the self-proclaimed World's Most Famous Arena. "It's kind of like the history here," Harrison said. "You see how many people have come through there and what they are doing now when you go to a place like that. When you have the opportunity to play in a place like that it gives you pride, and it humbles you. It gives you all of that."

Harrison needed her walking shoes that Saturday. A trip to New York City meant shopping expeditions for coaches and players, and Harrison was Johnson's shopping partner.

"Izzy is my younger version of me," Johnson said. "I bought her some heels, some pumps, they're like silvery glittery pumps. I think they are so cute and I got them for her for secret Santa day, and she loved them."

Johnson enlisted Shekinna Stricklen's help, and they set the shopping equivalent of screens for each other, along with scouting reports. "We had some people over here looking out and some people over here, saying, 'What's the price over there. They're lower over here.'"

Dean Lockwood isn't much of a shopper. He dresses impeccably and stylishly for games, but Lockwood tends to treat shopping as a purposeful function instead of as a leisure activity. "Whenever we went to New York there was always, always, always a shopping trip to Macy's. Pat hired a car, a black SUV," said Lockwood, who declined Summitt's invitation to join the staff and instead went for a run in Central Park. "They took them to Macy's, and remember this is Christmas. There are throngs of people everywhere."

Lockwood always carries his phone with him, and on this exercise excursion, a call came in from an area code of his home state of Michigan, but he didn't have the number programmed. "It is Tim Nash, who was the academic dean when I coached at Northwood University, and he is now vice president. He and his wife, Pam, are in New York." The couple had finished shopping and were trying to hail a cab when a black SUV pulled up to the curb. "Out gets Pat, and Tim loves Pat Summitt. Tim always thought a lot of me, but I went up three notches when Pat hired me. They are about to get in a cab, and he says, 'Pam, no, that's Coach Summitt over there. We will catch another cab.'"

Nash managed to get through the crowd to reach Summitt. "He comes up to her and he says, 'You're Pat Summitt.' He goes, 'I am Tim Nash. I worked with Dean Lockwood. I helped hire Dean at Northwood.' Rather than isn't that nice, good to meet you, she turns to everyone and says, 'It's Tim Nash. He knows Dean.' She brings Tim and his wife over to meet everybody and introduces them by name. I am sure Mickie and Holly are going, 'I want to get in that store. We could care less who knows Dean.'" Warlick laughed as she recalled the story. "She would talk to anybody on the street. People loved being around her."

"Tim, to this day, he thinks that was the biggest deal that Pat took the time to do that," Lockwood said. "He said, 'It's unbelievable how down to earth and gracious she was. She laughed with us and joked with us. She asked him, 'Did Dean stomp his foot like he does now?' He calls me and says, 'Lock, I just talked to your boss! She's right here.'"

The next day at the Garden, Tennessee dispatched DePaul 84–61 in the second game of the doubleheader for the Maggie Dixon Classic, which honors the late Maggie Dixon, the head coach of the United States Military Academy women's basketball team, who died unexpectedly of a heart condition in 2006. During the second half of the Baylor-St. John's game, the award was presented to Summitt at center court during a timeout with members of Dixon's family. Both benches stopped the timeout proceedings, and the players and coaches turned to face the court for the presentation. The Lady Vols had been in the locker room waiting for their game to start, but they slipped out to watch the ceremony. "It just shows that so many people respect Pat," Stricklen said. "People truly respect her and love her." The crowd gave Summitt a standing ovation, and included in its ranks were former Lady Vols Michelle Marciniak and Kara Lawson and Lawson's husband, Damien Barling, who ran a marathon in New York to raise money for Alzheimer's. The Northern California radio personality—D-Lo, as he was known on the air—and Lawson met in Sacramento when she played for the WNBA's Monarchs.

Lawson worked to raise money for the New York City chapter of the Alzheimer's Association. The news of the Lawson/Barling running team was tinged with some pre-announcement humor when Barling, falling back on his radio personality and marketing ability, issued a teaser via social media that the couple had some news. Online speculation was that Lawson was pregnant, and given the echo chamber effect of the Internet, the rumor spread quickly.

"I had friends and people in my family calling me and asking me and they actually knew what the announcement was," Lawson said. "I'm like, 'What are you talking about? You know what it is.' And they were like, 'Oh, OK.' I just found it pretty funny that people actually thought we would make an announcement like that on Facebook. That's not the way it's going to be announced if it does happen by teasing it on social media, that's for sure." Summitt laughed when told of how the initial announcement went a tad astray, but she noted, "I can't wait until they have a child. That will be great."

Baylor Coach Kim Mulkey and center Brittney Griner broke their time-out huddle in the Garden and hugged Summitt before she walked off the court. "I just told her I loved her," Mulkey said. "She means to the women's game what John Wooden means to the men's game. Her presence on that floor and what she means to all of us, I don't think that anybody will ever have that presence."

Meshia Thomas, a lieutenant with the UT Police Department, was close to Summitt as always. While her official title was with the UTPD, she was known as Summitt's bodyguard. Thomas hovered nearby—close but always out of the way, as she preferred—and waited to escort Summitt back to the locker room. Once they got off the court and into the back area of Madison Square Garden, Thomas saw something she had never seen in five years of walking with Summitt on game days: the coach had tears in her eyes. "I looked over at her and I could see her eyes were welled," Thomas said. "And I had never seen that. That was tough for me. She is always strong. I never saw a tear drop, just welled up. I said, 'Coach, you good?' She said, 'Yeah, that was hard.' And she just kept on."

Behind the pesky defense and timely offense of senior Alicia Manning, Tennessee was able to put away DePaul after letting a 12-point halftime lead dwindle to four within three minutes of the second half. Manning can always be counted on to crash the glass and play defense—she had 12 boards and four steals—but in the 84–61 win, she also contributed on offense with 12 points to complete the double-double.

Still, Massengale's absence was apparent from the opening tip, and Tennessee started the game with two consecutive turnovers. Meighan Simmons started at point guard but soon gave way to Shekinna Stricklen, who was better suited at small forward but remained a viable option at the top of the floor for Tennessee. "I was concerned about Meighan and the pressure that DePaul was putting on the point guard," Holly Warlick said. "We knew with Massengale out we would have to run the point guard by committee, and that's basically what we did. At times we had Taber bring the ball up a couple of times."

Stricklen settled down after a shaky start and played the bulk of her 34 minutes at the point position. She was particularly effective in the second half when she had zero turnovers. "Clearly, you can see in the first half I was thinking too much," Stricklen said. "Second half, Pat came up to me and said, 'Relax, play your game and you'll do fine.' I came out second half pushing the ball in transition, looking more for my teammates, and trying to get to the basket." DePaul could not stop Tennessee's repeated attacks at the rim and wore down well before the final buzzer.

That was the game plan for the Lady Vols. Warlick, who had the scout, said the intent was to get the ball to the paint either by entry passes or dribble drive. Tennessee attempted only five treys and missed each one. The last time Tennessee didn't connect on a three-pointer was against LSU in the SEC season opener on January 2, 2011. That game broke a streak of 422 consecutive games for Tennessee with a made three-pointer, but it was hardly noticeable this time around.

With the game in one of the country's major media markets in New York, the post-game press conference was crowded with media, and the players and Warlick were asked about Summitt, her disease, and its effect on the team. "I will tell you this: Pat Summitt is the coach at the University of Tennessee, and she is still coaching," Warlick said. "She has put the assistants in a unique situation where she has allowed us over the last three or four years to do the things she thinks we're best at. The sign of a great leader is to have a tremendous amount of support, and Pat relies on her support and she relies on the assistant coaches. It may be a little bit different, but she is still my boss. She is still leading us and still coaching this basketball team."

The questions were something the players were accustomed to by now, and their answers were script-like in their tendency to keep the focus on the court. The loss of Massengale was more troublesome to them; the second game of the road swing on December 13, 2011, would be much more difficult against a rugged Rutgers team with pesky and athletic guards. Rutgers deploys a trapping defense and extends its ball pressure 94 feet. Sure-handed guards are needed against the Scarlet Knights.

The last time the Lady Vols had traveled to Rutgers' arena, known as the RAC, Tennessee arrived with a team loaded with freshmen in the 2008–09 season. During the previous 2007–08 season, the Lady Vols had won 59–58 in Knoxville on two free throws by Nicky Anosike with .02 seconds left on the clock. For the rematch a year later, Scarlet Knight fans held up signs with clock images and asked what time it was, but there was surprisingly little rancor, and the crowd gave Summitt a standing ovation when she entered the athletic center. Such was the respect for Summitt on the road.

That January 3, 2009, game had started overwhelmingly in Rutgers' favor, and the Scarlet Knights led 33–13 at halftime, a record deficit for the Lady Vols midway through a game. "I remember we didn't score until seven minutes into the game and then going into halftime down by 20 and Pat going off and saying, 'I promise you, you don't want to go back on a plane with me if we lose this game,'" Stricklen said. The Lady Vols then proceeded to pull off the greatest comeback in program history with the 55–51 win. It surpassed the 17-point second-half deficit to Virginia in the regional finals of the 1996 NCAA Tournament, a game the Lady Vols won 52–46, advancing to beat Connecticut and Georgia in the Final Four in Charlotte, North Carolina, for Summitt's fourth national title.

"We made history from a bad way to a good way," Manning said. "I remember a hostile environment and I remember seeing a different side of our team that we hadn't seen before that—that heart and desire that we weren't going to give up." Manning and Stricklen were now seniors for this trip to Rutgers. The Lady Vols prevailed, 67–61, behind clutch three-point shooting from Stricklen, Simmons, and Spani and a pivotal block by Vicki Baugh late in the game. This time, the presence of Summitt was the most memorable part of the matchup.

Rutgers put out the welcome mat in 2011, from students selling Summitt's orange-and-purple "Fierce Courage" bracelets on the concourse to the scorer's table signage promoting her foundation to raise money for Alzheimer's to the Scarlet Knights wearing "We Back Pat" shooting shirts. As soon as the 6,368 fans in attendance saw Summitt coming around a corner of the stands with her team, they came to their feet with a sustained ovation and roar. The players were getting used to this, but Rutgers left an impression. "Rutgers sticks out right away to me," Spani said. "I feel like it was a five- to 10-minute standing ovation of the entire arena for Pat when she walked out."

The reaction elated Coach C. Vivian Stringer. "I am proud of them," Stringer said. "I wouldn't have expected anything less than that. I think the Scarlet Knight fans are classy people. . . . I know that Pat appreciated that." Stringer and her staff walked to Tennessee's bench, and when Stringer hugged Summitt, the applause somehow got even louder. "It was awesome," Warlick said. "It's just a tribute to the fans here and how they've appreciated Pat every year we've been up here. We knew the people in orange were going to stand up, but everyone in red . . . everybody in the whole arena was so positive, and Pat is so appreciative of that. It was a little overwhelming when we came out." After the game ended Summitt walked to the baseline, where Rutgers football player Eric LeGrand, who was paralyzed in a game in 2010, was waiting. The two spoke briefly, and that brought more appreciation from the fans who witnessed the exchange.

As the Lady Vols left the court, a pocket of Tennessee fans belted out "Rocky Top," and while they received some odd looks, there were no catcalls. A busload of fans had left Knoxville for the two-game road trip and certainly enjoyed their stay in the Northeast. "Obviously, I hope we can keep our momentum and keep it going and keep focused," Summitt said. "We are going to be back on the road real soon."

14

CALIFORNIA BOUND

The Lady Vols were home for one day in Knoxville before heading west for games against UCLA and Stanford. The players would scatter in different directions for Christmas break after the two games in California, so this trip involved commercial airlines rather than the usual charter flights for the Lady Vols' far-flung travels.

The team had a layover en route to Los Angeles and stopped at a Chili's restaurant for a meal. Airport restaurants typically have seating directly beside the concourse, and the Lady Vol players were sitting in that dining area of the Chili's both people-watching and being watched. "We were sitting down eating, but you can see people walk by, and, of course, we are wearing that bright orange," Vicki Baugh said. "He noticed, and he came up to our table, and we were like, 'Oh, my gosh.'"

The he in this case was Tim Hardaway, a five-time NBA All-Star whose No. 10 jersey was retired in 2009 by the Miami Heat. "He asked, 'Where's your coach?' Pat was sitting in the back of the restaurant. He went over to her table. He paid his respects to her, gave her a hug and was on his way. I just thought that was really cool. It shows you the impact that she had on sports."

The long day of travel to get to Los Angeles meant Strength & Conditioning Coach Heather Mason took over a ballroom at the team's Marina del Rey hotel for a stretching regimen to loosen up the players. The next morning, the Lady Vols were back on the practice court in UCLA's John Wooden Center, a quaint gymnasium with incredibly loose rims. Since Pauley Pavilion was in the midst of a major overhaul, the game would be played at the Wooden Center, which was the student recreation facility. In the span of a few days, the Lady Vols had gone from the bustle of the big city and Madison Square Garden to a small gym in a laid-back region of the country. "It's a little different," Holly Warlick said after that practice session ended. "I think this is like our Pratt Pavilion. I think we are comfortable here."

That was an understatement. The Lady Vols shot an eye-popping 76 percent in the first half, a program record, surpassing the 70.3 percent mark against Old Dominion on January 4, 1989. Tennessee then finished the game at a still-scorching 69.2 percent for an 85–64 win. "I wish I could say I was the shooting coach," Warlick joked after the game.

Summitt still talked to the media, especially in sessions back home in Knoxville, but Warlick handled all of the post-game press conferences in the 2011–12 season. Post-game events can sometimes be hurried in rooms with inadequate acoustics, and Tennessee didn't want to put Summitt on the spot—if she didn't hear a question or stumbled with an answer at any time, Tennessee knew that would be magnified. The endless loop of television sports shows and highlights meant that one slip-up could become a national and repeated event. If Summitt stumbled over her words in the season she had announced she had early onset dementia, the context, tone, and tenor of the situation would be utterly lost amid the endless repeat of her words.

The loss, ultimately, was to the game of basketball. Summitt could distill a game to its essence and usually tinged her remarks, win or lose, with wit and humor. She enjoyed the give and take with the media, and she was especially comfortable with the media in Knoxville, remaining so throughout her final season. When she became head coach emeritus, Summitt stopped and talked if she saw media members she had known for years. Openness with the media was as much a part of her legacy as wins and losses.

UCLA Coach Cori Close opened her remarks at the post-game press conference with a salute to Summitt. Her team was on a summer tour of

Italy in 2011 when Summitt's news was made public. "I will never forget it," Close said. "In our last night at Lake Como I talked about the things that we are benefiting from because of the trails that she has blazed. She set the standard."

Summitt always enjoyed the trips to California—yes, it meant another shopping excursion—and she had a great coaching relationship with Stanford's Tara VanDerveer. The Bay Area media also looked forward to the matchup, and several press members came to the Lady Vols' December 19 practice session on Stanford's campus in Palo Alto hoping to speak to Summitt. But she missed that Monday practice session because of a medical consultation appointment that had been scheduled for the West Coast trip. "She's fine," Warlick told the media. "It was something she wanted to go do."

Summitt was the topic of every road trip with a new set of reporters understandably following the storyline of a coach of her stature dealing with dementia. "I think when she found that out it was almost like a relief for her first off," Warlick said. "And then when she told everybody and made it public, that was a major burden off her shoulders, because she knew she couldn't hide something that was very personal to her. She wanted to make sure everybody knew, get it out there and let's move on. She's put a face on dementia. It's incredible. You have a face with that disease, and she's still working. She's amazing. Absolutely amazing. That's what she's done all her life. She's always put everything out there."

While the diagnosis was startling, to say the least, and crushing in the aftermath as Summitt tried to accept it, knowing exactly what was wrong also was some sort of relief. Summitt knew something was off, and she was frustrated. Warlick stepped to the forefront to handle the media, and she fielded a frequent question, especially on the road: how does the staff balance basketball duties with being the public face in the sport for Alzheimer's awareness? "I have learned to take one day at a time," Warlick said. "I think different days throw different things at me. I've learned so much from Pat, and I know she used to multitask so she forced all of us to multitask. I just go on her knowledge and her strength and hope my knowledge, what I've learned from her, has carried on and will continue to carry on with this team."

As the Lady Vols were leaving Stanford's practice facility to board the bus back to the team hotel, the Cardinal players were taking the court for their session. The Tennessee coaches stopped to chat with VanDerveer.

"We just have a tremendous amount of respect for Tara," Warlick said. "She runs a great program. She does things right."

The game before a sold-out crowd at Maples Pavilion on December 20, 2011, started in Tennessee's favor. The Lady Vols opened a 10–3 lead within the first three minutes and even boosted it to 16–7 at the 13:21 mark of the first half, despite the fact Vicki Baugh had left with her second personal foul at the 14:33 mark on what was called an illegal screen (a bizarre call that left Summitt and the coaching staff staring at the official in disbelief). Baugh can get in a funk when she gets into foul trouble, and this time she went into a deep one. She played just five minutes in the first half, and the Lady Vols lost their one post player with size, leaving the undersized Glory Johnson and Alicia Manning to try to handle the tall trees of Stanford.

A charging foul against Shekinna Stricklen in the first half that looked like an and-one play with the basket—a Stanford player was still bunny hopping into place when Stricklen arrived—was waved off, and an incredulous Summitt nearly walked to center court to challenge the call. Meanwhile, freshman Isabelle Harrison played a stretch of basketball she likely wants to purge from memory as she tossed an errant shot towards the rim and then went to the floor. She rose slowly and was at center court when Stanford, now playing five on four, scored an uncontested layup. At halftime Tennessee trailed by just seven points at 48–41, because neither team was playing much defense, and that continued throughout the second half.

The Lady Vols ultimately scored 80 points—usually enough to win any game—but Stanford scorched the nets for 97 with two Cardinal players posting career highs as Nneka Ogwumike tallied 42 points and Toni Kokenis, 26. The 97–80 loss ensured that the Christmas break would be a sour one for the Lady Vols. After a few minutes, VanDerveer entered the interview room and declared that Ogwumike had been "a woman with girls out there"—a remark that included players on both teams. Warlick had already had her turn with the media and had tried to explain what went awry against Stanford. A weary Warlick stood in the hallway and told two beat writers from Knoxville that defending one-on-one and ball pressure would top the priority list after Christmas break.

Warlick was gracious after the game; she saluted Ogwumike and noted that Tennessee played well in spurts but could not maintain any rhythm. She also correctly noted that the Lady Vols had been on the road for two weeks and had essentially not practiced. A coast-to-coast road trip means little time in the gym, and when the Lady Vols did take the court, it was for specific game preparation with a need to ensure the players had their legs. Indeed, the last time the Lady Vols had a full-court, full-scale practice was December 8, the day before they left for New York and the same day

Massengale dislocated a middle finger, causing her to miss three games on the road and enter in the second half against Stanford because the Lady Vols desperately needed someone to put pressure on the ball.

It had been a bizarre season in terms of hand and wrist injuries. Alicia Manning injured a thumb in preseason and was in a cast for a few weeks, Warlick broke her hand after SEC Media Day in a airport mishap, Massengale dislocated her finger trying to corral a loose ball, and Mickie DeMoss fractured her wrist the day before the Stanford game after someone stepped on her loose shoelace while the coaches walked to dinner (and right after Summitt had told her to stop and tie it). The pre-game storyline, of course, was Summitt. Stanford fans have long admired Summitt, and she received a sustained standing ovation when she walked onto the court. "I forget a lot of the time that she's Pat Summitt," Baugh said. "That was a wake-up call to me, seeing how much support that she got. I remembered this is *the* Pat Summitt."

The players, coaches and support staff dispersed for a holiday break with a 7–3 record. They would reconvene in Knoxville the day after Christmas to get ready for a game against Old Dominion on December 28 to close out 2011 and then get the SEC schedule started on January 1 at Auburn. The coaches had used the first 10 games of the season to get used to the new reality at Tennessee. Warlick had moved into more of a co-head coach role, and the staff and players were making adjustments. Summitt was less talkative during pre-game instruction with the team. She tended to be more vocal at halftime, but the players knew Summitt was measuring her words at times. "It was different than the first two years I was there," Taber Spani said. "She was holding back a little bit. You could tell she didn't want to make a mistake. It was just the onset of this horrible disease that was taking a toll on a woman that a lot of people looked at as invincible."

15
BACK TO WORK

Going into the holiday break with a loss always put a damper on Christmas for the coaching staff. Rather than focus on holiday festivities, coaches watch film. Warlick repeatedly queued up the Stanford game. "I watched it," she said, laughing when it was noted that was no way to spend Christmas. Warlick called Coach Pat Summitt over the break, and her mood was sour, too. That would soon change with a book presentation by Chamique Holdsclaw.

The Lady Vols ended 2011 with a home game against Old Dominion, and Alicia Manning entered the starting lineup at the behest of Summitt, who announced the change before tipoff. It surprised Manning, who rewarded her coach's faith with a career high of 15 rebounds. The head coach had to keep a tissue handy after the game, but she obviously wasn't watching film of the Lady Vols' 90–37 wipeout of the Monarchs. Summitt was reading tribute letters from former Lady Vols that had been bound into a book.

Holdsclaw spearheaded the project by contacting former players and asking them to jot down their thoughts about Summitt. The idea came to Holdsclaw following Summitt's announcement that she had early onset dementia. Holdsclaw didn't know what to say to Summitt, so she started writing about it in her journal. That prompted Holdsclaw to contact other players and managers who had spent time on Rocky Top, and the result was a book with photos of the players, who wrote about what Summitt had meant to them over the years. Holdsclaw presented the book to Summitt at a team gathering before the Old Dominion tipoff.

When Summitt arrived for the standard pre-game meal with her team, she saw a crowded dining area. "I thought, 'Well, something is going on,'" Summitt said. At least 20 former Lady Vols were in attendance, including Sidney Spencer (2003–07), Michelle Marciniak (1993–96), Cindy Boggs (1974–75), and Carla McGhee (1986–90). Summitt scanned the book during the presentation and then read it closely once she got home. "It's phenomenal," she said, teary-eyed. "The book is unbelievable. It is special that they put all this together. It really touched my heart."

Holdsclaw, who won three national titles at Tennessee, has also endured her share of personal trials with the unexpected death of the grandmother who raised her and a battle with severe depression that drove her to a suicide attempt. "Chamique put this whole thing together," Summitt said. "We have a great relationship. She's reached out to me in a lot of different ways. She's been the one that rallied all the troops and had everybody there." The team went out and played as if they wanted Summitt to have time afterwards to read the letters rather than fret over breakdowns on the game film. Tennessee dominated in every category in the box score from rebounds (54 to 32) to points in the paint (46 to 8) to assists (26 to 8) to steals (16 to 3) to points off turnovers (26 to 1) to bench points (34 to 4).

Manning assisted on the highlight play of the game late in the second half. She got the defensive board and passed ahead to Briana Bass, who went behind the back with the right hand to Cierra Burdick, who went behind the back with the left hand to Manning, who was trailing the play. Manning hit the layup and ended up sprawled on the baseline after the foul as the Lady Vols bench erupted in celebration. She hit the free throw to complete the three-point play with 44 seconds remaining in the game.

Ariel Massengale also returned and immediately showed how much she had been missed during a play very early in the game. The ball was on the right side of the court, and Manning had popped free on the baseline on the left side, her arm up calling for the ball. Massengale, who didn't have the ball yet, was on the opposite baseline but saw Manning with a quick glance. She headed to the top of the court, got the ball from the wing, drove to pull the defense to her, which had sagged a bit to the basket, and fired the ball across the paint to Manning, who stuck the baseline shot.

Warlick, a former Lady Vol point guard, could not help but smile when she talked about Massengale. "She knows who to give the ball to at the right time," Warlick said. When Summitt had announced that Massengale— a Bolingbrook, Illinois, high school teenager at the time—would start at Tennessee, Warlick had said to wait and watch and then it would make sense. During the post-game press conference, Old Dominion Coach Karen Barefoot saluted Summitt for something that had happened nearly 20 years previously.

Old Dominion had been a powerhouse with some epic battles against Tennessee. The Lady Vols' fifth national title came against Old Dominion in 1997, a hard-fought 68–59 win in Cincinnati. In 2011, Barefoot was in her debut season as the Monarchs' head coach with a goal of returning the school to the national spotlight. When she started out in the profession, Barefoot wrote a letter to Summitt. "Seventeen years ago when I was 22 years old, I had an opportunity to be a young head coach, a college coach, and didn't know what to do and I wrote a letter to her not thinking I would get a response," Barefoot said. "She wrote back saying all these positive things and for me, to play here and play against her, thank you isn't enough to say for what she has done for me. She really gave me a positive message saying to go out there and teach and be a life coach and that changed my life."

Tennessee coaches divide the season into three distinct parts: non-conference games, SEC play, and postseason. The Lady Vols were about to embark on the SEC slate with a road game at Auburn on New Year's Day. "Could we have been better than our 8–3 record heading into conference play?" Summitt asked. "Probably. But right now we have to move forward and focus on what is coming up in the SEC."

The Lady Vols would lead by just two points at halftime in Auburn, Alabama, and Summitt had quite a bit to say to her players during the break in the locker room. "Basically if we don't get it together, then we're walking home," Glory Johnson said of Summitt's message. "And it's a long walk."

The Lady Vols quickly stretched the lead to 40–29 to start the second half—Tennessee would ultimately win, 73–52—and Auburn called timeout. Before joining her assistant coaches, Summitt went to the huddle and spoke emphatically to her players. She still had a powerful effect on them. They needed to hear her voice, and at the same time, her assistant coaches had to adjust depending on what was best for her. "Holly deserves such great credit," Dean Lockwood said. "Here is this person she played for, idolizes, respected, was mentored by her, for 27 years she was her right-hand lieutenant and now there are times when she has to assert herself and step in."

Still, Summitt could seize control of the situation when she felt the team needed her voice and commanding presence. "Her passion never waned at all, never dissipated," Lockwood said. "There were moments she wanted to make sure this team didn't feel shortchanged by her condition. She would dig to get that old Pat, maybe even be heavier-handed in moments when it would catch you, like, wow. There were times when she needed Holly to be more of a voice. But there were also times when she felt like, 'They need to hear my voice.' The true champion in Pat and the passion and the deep love that she has for this game came out. She felt like, 'I have to give these kids my best. This is my team, and they need me.'"

The Lady Vols were about to enter the grind of the SEC (though they had two non-conference games sprinkled in against Chattanooga on January 3 in Knoxville and Notre Dame on January 23 in South Bend), and the season, as always, would become a blur of practice, scouting, travel, rinse and repeat.

Tennessee handled Chattanooga with ease, 90–47, a game that was more memorable because it marked the return of junior Kamiko Williams, who had torn her ACL over the summer. With Taber Spani dealing with a deep bone bruise in her knee that limited her availability (she missed nine games that season), Williams was much-needed on the perimeter. Williams' first two years on campus were a major adjustment for a player who had never been asked to play defense in high school and who wasn't used to having teammates on the floor who could contribute. Her directive in high school was to score. Needless to say, Williams and Summitt clashed quite a bit as Summitt tried to keep the parts of Williams' game that worked well (driving ability, shot creation) and shed the ones that didn't (porous defense, a tendency to play by herself).

Williams listened and learned, and then she got hurt that summer and was at a crossroads. A player still in the process of shedding bad court habits would not top anyone's list of ideal rehab candidates. But Williams plunged into the process and worked as hard as anyone ever has at Tennessee. She earned Summitt's respect—Summitt tore her ACL in college and had to rehab to get ready for the 1976 Olympics—and Williams likely discovered a reservoir of desire for the game that she had never had to tap into before because basketball had come so easily for her. "It was good to see Kamiko back out on the floor," Summitt said. "She has worked so hard coming back from her torn ACL."

Cierra Burdick provided the final fireworks in the romp over Chattanooga. She tracked a long rebound to the sideline and knocked the ball off a Lady Moc before slamming into Lockwood on the bench, just missing Warlick. "Dean is learning to jump in my path so I won't get injured," Warlick said. "I'm just glad she didn't hit Pat. If she took Dean or me out and didn't hit Coach Summitt, we're in business." Meanwhile, it was another high-voltage game for Johnson, who energized her teammates with a block in the first half. A teammate leaned the wrong way on a backdoor cut, and the Lady Moc had what seemed like an utterly uncontested layup. But Johnson sprinted from the opposite side and sent the ball emphatically in the other direction. "Glory knew she had the talent, and Pat knew she had the talent, but if Pat didn't give her that extra oomph, I feel like Glory wouldn't have had that extra fire her senior year," Simmons said.

Georgia was the first SEC opponent at home for Tennessee, and Summitt, Lockwood, and Warlick addressed the Big Orange Tipoff Club the day before the game. The club meets at the landmark Calhoun's restaurant on the Tennessee River, a long pass from Neyland Stadium and popular dock spot for the Vol Navy, the fleet of boats that arrive for Tennessee football games every fall.

Former Lady Vol Abby Conklin, whose epic clashes with Summitt were part of the HBO documentary on the Lady Vols program, was a surprise visitor to the locker room before the Chattanooga game Conklin also attended Summitt's speech at the Tipoff Club, where she acknowledged her former player and had Conklin stand to be recognized. "I was never close to her as a player, but she is someone that I respect tremendously and as you get further away from being in the program you really see the impact that she had on your life."

Summitt was in excellent form at the Tipoff Club, telling jokes about tripping DeMoss on the road, talking in detail about her team, and taking questions from the audience. Anyone who walked in that room would not have thought that the woman speaking had dementia. Her speech was interrupted when a fan fell out of his chair. "Oops, are you all right?" Summitt said. "He must be a part of our staff because we are all falling down, too."

A fan asked Summitt, "Not a pleasant subject, Pat, but could you comment about the Stanford game and those two sisters?" Summitt feigned disgust about the Ogwumike sisters and said, "Did you have to bring that up?"

The fan: "They were unbeatable."

Summitt deadpanned: "I know. We watched. I was there."

Lockwood interjected with an anecdote to underscore the popularity of Summitt in a story he had never publicly told. He reminded the attendees about the time Summitt confronted a raccoon on her back porch that was menacing her beloved Labrador retriever, Sally Sue. The confrontation happened right before the SEC Tournament in 2008, and Summitt dislocated her shoulder knocking the raccoon off the railing. "We are in that little stretch that is in between the SEC Tournament and the NCAA Tournament," Lockwood said. "I am working late. I am doing some video at the office. I am driving home and I pull into a station a little bit after midnight. I need to fill up. I am running on fumes. At that time of night it pays to be aware of your surroundings. I see this guy at the next pump over. I have my Tennessee sweats and gear on and this guy is looking at me. He is kind of a rough-looking guy. He is close to my age, and he keeps looking over at me as he is pumping gas. He says, 'Hey, you're that man fellow with the Lady Vols.' I am looking at his car, and there is a gun rack in the back of the truck. I am trying to think of an exit. He said, 'You work every day with Coach Summitt, don't you? You see her every day, don't you?'"

By now, Warlick and Summitt, like everyone in attendance, were laughing out loud.

"He walks over a little closer and now I am really getting ready to leave. He has something in his hand and he says, 'Will you give her this for me?' And it's got his name and a phone number. And he says, 'That's my kind of woman right there. Any woman that's going to square off and tangle with a raccoon, that's my kind of woman. I'd like to meet her!' I thought discretion was the better part of valor and I've never said anything up until now."

Lockwood got a high-five from Summitt as he left the podium.

16

HEALING POWER OF HUMOR

Pat Summitt has a wicked sense of humor and a comedian's sense of timing.

Summitt also enjoyed interacting with the news media. She opened her practice sessions to the press and the public and made sure reporters who covered the team had her home and cell phone numbers. During a preseason workout one fall, two rather ragged-looking reporters—in other words, standard dress for the beat—walked into Pratt Pavilion to get Summitt's early take on the team. The *News Sentinel's* Dan Fleser was in shorts, sandals, and a T-shirt that looked plucked off the top of the laundry pile. The other reporter was in jeans with a collared but untucked shirt that had never seen an iron—that would be me from *InsideTennessee*. Summitt, who was always impeccably attired on the sideline and neatly dressed at practice, eyed both with a wry grin. When told it was part of a writer's charm to dress in such a way, Summitt cocked her head and said, "Oh, really?" When told the wrinkled shirt came from a $3 sale rack, Summitt replied, "You overpaid."

"There were great laughs being around her," said Meshia Thomas, the UT police officer who was so often by her side. "She enjoyed people. She would get that little smile on her face and shake that head. She was a ham. She could cut up." Summitt's sense of humor was a godsend for her team after the diagnosis. It lightened moments and kept the players loose. It also showed them that Summitt was dealing with her disease in the same way she had taught her players to handle life: accept it and keep going.

"I think Pat had a whole different perspective on the game and a whole different perspective on life," Mickie DeMoss said. "She didn't take things quite as seriously. She found more humor in stuff than she had in the past. She honestly seemed a little lighter. A little more I don't want to say carefree but not as burdened with wins and losses and the program. She had life in a better perspective." DeMoss was going over a scouting report in practice and noticed the players were starting to smile. Summitt had picked up DeMoss' glasses from the scorer's table and was standing behind her with the glasses perched on her nose. "The kids were laughing and Mickey turned around and Pat would go, 'Who am I?'" Holly Warlick said. "You just start laughing."

Meighan Simmons remembers walking into practice with Glory Johnson, Kamiko Williams, and Shekinna Stricklen and seeing Summitt holding a basketball. "Sometimes in practice I have a tendency to palm a ball," Simmons said. "It was me, Glory, Miko, and Strick coming in, and she saw me. She stood up and palmed the ball, and she was like, 'Who am I?' Glory looked at me and started dying laughing. She said, 'That's Meigh. All day.' It was things like that that we knew she still had some extra joy in her. She hadn't lost her way. She still had a way to have peace of mind with where she was at. She found some way to bring joy to us. We didn't have to be so emotionally worn out about this illness."

During one particular pre-practice huddle, Ariel Massengale recalls Summitt getting distracted by DeMoss' shoes. "I am standing next to Pat and she whispers in my ear, 'Look at Mickie. She's got on two different shoes,'" Massengale said. "I am trying to hold in my laugh because I think Mickie or Holly was talking. And then Pat said, 'What did she do? Get dressed in the dark this morning?' I just busted out laughing." DeMoss called out the freshman for laughing in the huddle, and Massengale shared Summitt's observation. "She looked down and had no idea she had on two different shoes," Massengale said. "She did actually get dressed in the dark. And it was probably the funniest thing ever."

Summitt was always in demand during her tenure at Tennessee. Her calendar, maintained by longtime secretary Katie Wynn, looked like a game of Twister writ small with color-coded entries covering every day. But in Summitt's final season, she would smile and tell her staff that she finally had an out. "She talked about a number of times it's great now because I can tell people, 'You know I don't remember that. I have dementia. I can be very selective. If I don't want to do something, I can tell them I forgot about it,'" Dean Lockwood said. "She said it good-naturedly."

Tyler Summitt, a senior at Tennessee during his mother's last season, was a frequent visitor to the basketball office. He served as a practice player one season for the Lady Vols and was a walk-on for the Vols basketball team for two seasons under Bruce Pearl and then Cuonzo Martin. He earned a bachelor's degree in just three years and did so summa cum laude in the UT Chancellor's Honors Program. Needless to say, his days and nights were filled. "I would walk in the office and say, 'Dang, where are my keys?'" Tyler said. "Mom goes, 'Now, Tyler, you know I'm the one with dementia, not you.'"

Thomas provided security for Pat as she had done for so many years, including at Tyler's wedding. Anywhere Summitt went, people wanted to talk to her. Thomas expected to keep an eye on matters in the background, but the wedding party members wanted Thomas with them. "They insisted I come back with the family," Thomas said. The wedding photos were to be taken in a nearby cemetery, so Thomas accompanied Summitt on the walk from the church. That meant navigating some stone steps and moving around tombstones, all while being approached by guests who wanted to talk to the coach. Thomas needed to deliver Summitt safely to the photo location, where the bride, groom, and families were assembling. "I said, 'Coach, this is not a good time to be falling. Watch these tombstones,'" Thomas said. Summitt came to a stop, looked at Thomas and said, "Who would take wedding pictures in a cemetery?'"

That sense of humor served Summitt and her staff well during her final season. While Tennessee was always a national contender, the Lady Vols hadn't been to a Final Four since 2008 for an assortment of reasons, with a brutal run of injuries topping the list. The pressure to break that drought arrived with the start of every season, and the 2011–12 squad with five seniors especially felt a sense of urgency. Now those players also had the pressure of knowing they could be Summitt's last team. Tennessee overall held up well throughout the season, but the Lady Vols fell apart in South Bend on a bitterly cold evening January 23, 2012, and lost 72–44.

"They were beating us pretty bad in the second half," DeMoss said. "I looked at Pat and said, 'Well, maybe they can just let the clock run.' She said, 'Yeah, that wouldn't be bad, would it?' Clearly, the game was out of hand. We didn't have a chance to win and I would have never said that to her before. After I said that I thought, 'Wow, I can't believe I said that.'" The Notre Dame fans erupted in cheers and held signs aloft in support when Summitt took the court before the game, and Summitt had been very vocal during that game, but she had a keen sense of perspective that season. "Her humor throughout the process really helped," Jenny Moshak said. "She was serious when it was time to be serious, but I think some of her perspectives on things were starting to change."

After the team returned to Knoxville from South Bend, the media had access to conduct interviews and get practice video. Summitt, as she was wont to do, approached a sportswriter on the sideline to briefly chat.

"What did you think of the game?" Summitt asked.

"That was brutal," I replied.

"I don't remember it," Summitt said, and she walked back to the court smiling.

17

SEC SEASON

After the win over Auburn on the road to start 2012, the Lady Vols opened the SEC slate at home against Georgia. The Lady Vols had gone 16–0 in the SEC during the 2010–11 season and won the 2011 tournament in Duluth, Georgia, with wipeouts of Florida, Georgia, and Kentucky. The last loss to an SEC team was against Georgia in Athens on January 21, 2010, a three-point defeat during a 15–1 campaign in the 2009–10 season that also included an SEC tourney crown.

On January 29, 2012, the Lady Vols ran their streak of SEC wins to 35 with an 80–51 wipeout of a ranked Georgia team. Sophomore Meighan Simmons had, to this point, never lost an SEC game in her career. "I can tell you I didn't see this coming," Pat Summitt said after that game. "Georgia is a very good basketball team, but we just came out and executed for 40 minutes. Across the board, everyone stepped up and contributed. It was a good team win, and I am proud of how we played." It was an indication of how well Tennessee could play, though in a little more than two weeks, the

Lady Vols would play like a shell of themselves against the aforementioned Notre Dame.

The Lady Vols were on the road for the next two games with trips to Arkansas and Kentucky. The contest in Arkansas was always a family reunion for Shekinna Stricklen, who is from the small town of Morrilton, and a busload of family and friends arrived in Fayetteville to see the home state star. Some players get uptight during these types of homecoming games, but Stricklen never did. She always played better in front of family, and she did so in Arkansas with 19 points and eight rebounds.

On January 8, 2012, Arkansas was outmatched from the opening tip: the Lady Vols started the game with an 11–0 run and shot 50 percent overall from the field. The only good statistic in the box score for the Razorbacks was the 93.8 percent marksmanship from the line. Tennessee demolished Arkansas 69–38. "Let's talk about our free throw shooting," Arkansas Coach Tom Collen quipped afterwards, before noting, "We were totally outplayed from beginning to end." Summitt preached a mantra of playing a 40-minute game, and the team has been inching closer to playing in her image. "I think we're progressing in that direction each and every day," Summitt said on her post-game radio show. "This team, as I have said before, really wants to win."

Stricklen's teammates sometimes teased her about the influx of family and friends–they tend to arrive en masse—"but my teammates love my family," she said. Stricklen had been home twice before the game—for the Christmas holidays and earlier in the season after the death of her maternal grandfather, James Moore.

"He made us laugh," Stricklen said. "He could never say my name right so he always called me Tina. He could never say Kinna."

On January 12, 2012, the SEC streak came to an end in Lexington on an evening when snow fell, temperatures dipped well below freezing, and parking lots iced over. Still, that didn't stop more than 8,000 fans from getting to Memorial Coliseum, and they watched a raucous celebration on the court after Kentucky nipped Tennessee, 61–60, while the Lady Vols huddled for their post-game prayer. Among the celebrants was Kyra Elzy, a former Lady Vol and Kentucky native who had been a tremendous recruiter for Kentucky as an assistant coach. She was as responsible for that win over Tennessee as anyone on the staff. A year later, Elzy would be summoned home, as it were, by Holly Warlick, who was putting together her first staff as a head coach and needed proven assistants to keep Pat Summitt's legacy on a Tennessee track.

Elzy walked into the Kentucky basketball complex to find her office packed, a rather rude reaction, especially to a coach who had done so much for the Wildcats. In comparison, when then-Auburn Coach Nell Fortner learned Daedra Charles-Furlow would leave the Tigers' staff in 2008 for a spot on Summitt's sideline, she hugged Charles-Furlow and told her she understood when a coach returned to her alma mater, especially to a program like Tennessee's. Packing an assistant's office in the absence of firing or malfeasance wasn't well received, to say the least, and the tension between the Tennessee and Kentucky staffs went from simmering to ablaze.

The relationship ultimately was repaired. In 2016, Elzy left Tennessee and returned to Kentucky as Mitchell replaced his entire staff.

Elzy's Kentucky bio lauded her as a top recruiter and credited her with helping to bring a top-10 recruiting class to Lexington for three straight seasons, including the signing of four high school McDonald's All-Americans. The bio also described A'dia Mathies as one of "Elzy's guards" who had received SEC recognition. In that game against Tennessee, Mathies torched the Lady Vols for 34 points and lofted the game winner with 4.2 seconds left. "She has been very good in those situations and that's why recruiting is so important," Kentucky Coach Matthew Mitchell said. "That was not a real genius coaching move right there. That was a great player making a big-time play. That's the formula. That's how Tennessee has won so many games over the years—players making great plays. We did a good day's work when we signed A'dia Mathies."

The Wildcats fans erupted when Summitt walked onto the court before the game, and a pack of photographers swarmed the Tennessee bench to get closer as Mitchell and Summitt greeted each other. "I tell Pat before every game that I wouldn't be out here without what she did," said Mitchell, who was once a camp worker and graduate assistant for Tennessee. "I really appreciate our fans tonight. They did exactly what first-class people should do." The photographers ended up behind and in front of the bench. Tennessee's players weaved around them to get to the pre-game huddle, another example of the refuge of the court being compromised that season.

Summitt had plenty to say during the game to the officials, who called a style that the Wildcats need with their swarming defense—if a lot of whistles blow with contact, the defense is not very effective. Tennessee's posts were hacked at the rim while shooting and rebounding, and the guards had escorts who clutched handfuls of uniforms as they tried to make their cuts. Ariel Massengale was called for a travel after being taken down because the defender had the front of her jersey knotted in her hand.

Glory Johnson adjusted in the second half by ripping away rebounds, which the fans didn't like, but she had smaller guards trying to snatch the ball. Her aggressiveness worked, as they backed off. Just before Mathies' game winner, with 28 seconds left and Tennessee up by one, Stricklen drove to the paint and was called for an offensive foul. Tennessee's bench howled in protest, and Summitt, who had a straight-on view of the play, was livid on the sideline. But the Lady Vols had started slow in the first half, gone down by 12 late in the second half, and blamed themselves for the loss. "A lot of us just put on the jersey and think that's what it's going to take, but it takes a lot more hard work on every possession," Vicki Baugh said.

Tennessee headed home with a shot to redeem themselves: a January 15, 2012, matchup with bitter in-state rival Vanderbilt. The Lady Vols started the game as if Kentucky were still on their minds, and Summitt had to deliver the thunder at halftime. "She challenged them the way Pat Summitt challenges them," Warlick said. "They were inspired when they left the locker room."

"She asked us, 'What have we been doing? This looks like the Kentucky game,'" Baugh said. "We're wearing 'We Back Pat' shirts as well. We know we're Tennessee, and we can't just put on the orange and win. I think she reinforced that." The entire week of home games in the SEC, women and men, was part of the "We Back Pat" initiative in which schools promote Summitt's foundation and raise awareness of Alzheimer's. Tennessee's assistant coaches donned their usual dress suits, but with a fashion twist: they wore "We Back Pat" T-shirts with their suit jackets. Summitt sported an orange blazer that she often breaks out for the Vandy game, but she didn't wear her own T-shirt underneath it.

The first half wasn't Summitt's style of basketball. The second half was vintage Tennessee. "It doesn't hurt to remind them about the pride of wearing the orange . . . especially when you are playing your cross-state rival in Vanderbilt," Summitt said. "I think they received the message I delivered and responded in a positive way." The defensive issues in the first half started on the ball, and Vandy's guards got little resistance from Ariel Massengale, Meighan Simmons, and Shekinna Stricklen.

"It started with Ariel on the ball," Warlick said. "When she had pressure, Shekinna got more intense, Meighan got more intense, and it carried over." The team responded with inspired defense in the second half to transform a three-point game at halftime into a 23-point victory, 87–64, before a thunderous home crowd of 17,879. The victory was Summitt's 500th win at home.

The game was also a showcase for Johnson, who had vowed to leave Tennessee with no regrets caused by not playing hard on every possession. If hu-

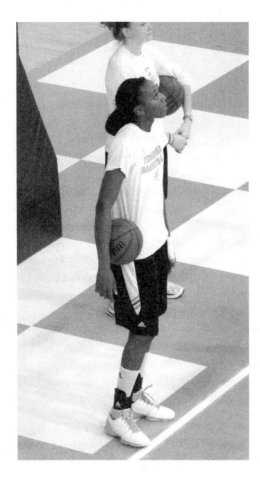

Glory Johnson was rarely without a basketball in hand during the final season. She wanted to leave with no doubt about how hard she worked.

man cloning were truly possible, the Lady Vols likely would have duplicated Johnson. Since the loss at Stanford, Johnson played with a combination of ferocity and poise at both ends of the floor, and she did so despite absorbing a physical beating in every game. In post-game press conferences, she looked like a human Popsicle with ice bags taped to assorted body parts. "Glory is our rock," Warlick said. "If we have to lay our hat on somebody, it's Glory Johnson."

Before the game, Johnson stood with Summitt at center court to be honored with a ceremonial game ball to recognize the fact that she became the fourth player in program history to score at least 1,000 points and tally at least 1,000 rebounds. The other three were Sheila Frost, Chamique Holdsclaw, and Tamika Catchings. Summitt and Johnson posed for photos, and before Johnson ran to the tunnel for pre-game introductions, Summitt hugged the senior forward and told Johnson that she loved her. "She did," Johnson said. "It means so much. She's been taking care of me since I got here as a freshman. She's always had my back, even when she's yelling at me." Johnson smiled as she walked away from her coach and then went out and played Summitt's style of basketball against Vanderbilt—a team Summitt always wanted to beat. "Glory just plays so hard," Summitt said. "You probably noticed it was pretty physical in there. I was really impressed with Glory's composure and energy."

One play in particular summed up Johnson's approach to the season. In the first half she was the only defender putting pressure on the guards, so Tennessee had to shift her out of the paint despite Vandy's size. She deflected the ball away from a Vandy ball handler, and the ball bounced toward center court. The Vandy player was now between Johnson and the ball, and the easy thing to do would have been to reset and await the ball again. But Johnson darted around the Commodore, dove for the ball, secured it for Tennessee, and got her head driven into the court when the Vandy player—perhaps startled that Johnson had scooted past her—dove onto her back.

While Jenny Moshak attended to Johnson and then helped her walk to the bench, Summitt summoned one of the officials, pointed to the spot on the floor, and stated her case. The crowd erupted with applause, and fans gave Summitt a standing ovation. Johnson spent the final 1:49 of the first half with an ice pack on her eye, and resilient as she was, she was back on the court for the start of the second half. Her impact was such that the opposing team's scheme was to steer the ball away from her. "We try to avoid entering the ball when she is defending and have our other post come up and give us some relief," Vanderbilt Coach Melanie Balcomb said. "She makes it difficult for you to enter the ball to the post to start your offense, as well as anytime you set a ball screen. If she is the one out hedging or trapping hard, she's really tough on getting deflections. She is so athletic on smaller guards like we have."

The only downside for Tennessee in the game was a late exit by Stricklen, who collided with a Commodore going for a rebound and injured her knee. The good news came the next day that the injury was a knee sprain that would hinder her day-to-day performance and not a torn ACL that would have ended her season. The sense of relief was etched all over Stricklen's face. She had had to wait until the afternoon for an MRI appointment. "I am thinking I am going to do it that morning, and I texted Jenny, and she was like, '3:20.' I was like, 'Are you serious?' So, I do it and then went an hour, and I am sitting by my phone constantly (checking) and like, 'When is she going to call? When is she going to call?' Finally she called and she said, 'It's not your ACL.' And I said, 'That's all I need to hear.' I just sat there and thanked God so many times. It clearly opened my eyes not to take a game for granted."

Tennessee had another home test against LSU—matchups with the Tigers tended to be close games—and the day before felt like a family reunion with two former Lady Vols on the LSU staff. Nikki Caldwell, a native of nearby Oak Ridge, Tennessee, was in her first season as LSU's head coach, and Tasha Butts had followed Caldwell from UCLA to Baton Rouge as an assistant. LSU practiced right after Tennessee did on 'The Summitt' court. In addition, Tony Perotti, an LSU assistant coach, was a Lady Vol practice player from 1997 to 1999, while former Angel Elderkin, who was the Lady Vols' video coordinator from 2005 to 2007, served LSU in the same capacity that season.

When Caldwell arrived at the arena, both staffs greeted each other with hugs and smiles. The friendly socialization would give way the following evening when both benches wanted to win a basketball game. "She probably feels like she knows us better than a lot of other teams," Summitt said. "But that's OK. We know her. She knows us. We've got to go play." Warlick added, "She called during practice and I answered and she goes, 'What are you doing?' I said, 'We're trying to get ready for you.' She said, 'If you don't have it down by now, you're in trouble.'" The January 19, 2012, game was played without Stricklen, who was nursing that knee sprain, and Taber Spani, who was still being held out because of the bone bruise in her knee.

When the Lady Vols and Lady Tigers tangle, it tends to get physical in the paint. This time, the battle extended to every inch of the court. The game was a grind that saw two Lady Tigers knocked out before halftime—one with a concussion within the first two minutes—and Glory Johnson sent to the locker room with a shoulder injury before the half ended. "You saw two teams really playing every possession like it was their last," Caldwell said.

Freshman Cierra Burdick knew this SEC rivalry was traditionally a hard-fought one, but it exceeded her expectations. The day before the game, Summitt had mentioned Burdick as one of the players who would need to step up because of the depleted roster. "It was more than what I thought," Burdick said. "Players were hitting the deck every single possession, but we came out to play. That's exciting. People want to see that. People want to come and pay money and see women just battle on the floor. I think we did a great job of that, and I hope our fans approve." The 13,107 in attendance did indeed, when not in a full-throated roar directed at the officials. Summitt stomped and screamed over the calls and non-calls while Caldwell, sporting

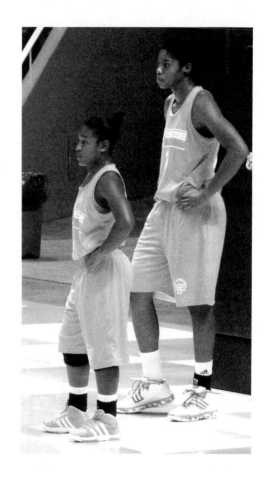

Briana Bass and Vicki Baugh played for Pat Summitt during that final season and became close friends.

high heels and seven months pregnant with her first child, did the same on her end of the court.

"They just battled," Warlick said. "I wouldn't expect anything less by a team coached by Nikki or a team coached here." LSU lost guard Jeanne Kenney early in the first half after she took an elbow to the eye. She was diagnosed with a concussion and didn't return. Then, with less than four seconds to play before halftime, Lady Vol Briana Bass picked up LSU's Destini Hughes deep in the backcourt when LSU in-bounded the ball under Tennessee's basket. Hughes bolted for the other end, and Bass ran into a screen, taking her out of the play for the moment.

The long in-bounds pass was intended for Hughes with Vicki Baugh and Isabelle Harrison, who were back for Tennessee, also leaping for the ball as it hung in the air. Hughes came down with the ball, and her right leg crumpled underneath her and bent at an awkward angle. Bass, who had caught up with the play, slid around her to avoid contact. The injury occurred in front of Tennessee's bench, and both Summitt and Caldwell went to the fallen player. A senior guard, Hughes stayed down for several minutes while medical personnel from both teams came to her aid. Inflatable casts were used to stabilize the leg, and Hughes left the floor in a wheelchair with several Lady Vol players patting her on the head. It was later determined that her knee was shredded, ending her season.

Minutes before that play, Johnson injured her shoulder on the other end in a scramble for a loose ball that had been batted around and was up in the air. She was taken to the locker room for the remainder of the first half. "I just saw the ball, I went up and I kind of tried to get it with both hands, and I think one of my shoulders (got) knocked back, and I heard a pop, and that's when I was holding it," said Johnson, who dislocated the same shoulder in practice two years previously. The coaches didn't know at halftime if Johnson would be cleared to play. Wearing a thick brace, she ran onto the court from the Lady Vols locker room seconds before the second half started. She took a seat on the bench, and Burdick started in her place. "She was in a lot of pain at halftime," Warlick said. "She was back in the training room. I wasn't sure, then Jenny came up and said she could go. That was part of Glory being competitive and a tough-minded kid. We needed her. We needed her to step up, and she did."

It also was a breakout game for Burdick on both ends of the court. The freshman went the distance in the second half in what seems to always be the toughest SEC matchup of the regular season in terms of player collisions. "I thought Cierra played her best game," Summitt said. "She showed a lot of poise, and her 15 points and six rebounds off the bench were pretty big for us." Tennessee prevailed, in every sense of the word, with a 65–56 win.

Two days later the Lady Vols departed for South Bend, Indiana, ready to see how they would measure up against Notre Dame—the game in which Summitt ended up wryly agreeing to the notion of a running clock—and the team that had knocked Tennessee out of the NCAA Tournament in 2011. The Fighting Irish were ranked No. 2 in the country and apparently had a chip on their shoulders thanks to a comment in the Lady Vols' game notes.

18

TRIP TO SOUTH BEND

Tennessee had dominated the Notre Dame series for years. The Fighting Irish had come close on several occasions but the Lady Vols had a 20–0 slate until 2011 in the Elite Eight game. Game notes are prepared for all matchups by media relations departments across the country in all sports. The Lady Vols' notes mentioned the "luck of the Irish"—an oft-used and well-known phrase that dates to the second half of the nineteenth century—in breaking the losing streak to Tennessee. The phrase has taken on a common meaning of good fortune, but its roots trace to overcoming a difficult situation. In either context, it was benign.

But coaches are always looking for ways to motivate their teams, and Notre Dame's Muffet McGraw used those four words among thousands in the game notes to rankle her team and imply the last win was no more than luck. After the game, a local columnist who was aware of the gamesmanship asked McGraw about "luck," and she smiled. The rest of the media was initially confused, but the context was revealed in the press conference.

The Lady Vols arrived in South Bend on January 22, 2012, to snow and bitterly cold temperatures. South Bend is not a destination of choice in late January, and the Lady Vols were far from healthy. Taber Spani had been rehabbing her knee since Christmas break and remained a game-day decision. At Saturday's practice two days before the game, Glory Johnson wore the thick black brace to protect her left shoulder. She spent the team's off day on Friday getting three hours of rehab with Jenny Moshak. Teammate Alicia Manning could sympathize; she had the side of her face clawed in a 2011 game against the Lady Tigers, so she was happy to emerge unscathed.

"I was like, 'Man, I am so glad it's not me this time,'" Manning said. "It was a rough one. Usually I'm the one that gets the brunt of it, but Glory has been getting hammered lately." Manning and Johnson had attended the Lady Vols' Salute to Excellence gala on Friday evening, an annual event of support and fundraising for the women's sports programs that later became for all UT athletics, and, perhaps not coincidentally, was not as well attended as when it focused on the Lady Vols. Seniors represent the various teams at the event, and sleeveless gowns are often the dress of choice for the student-athletes. "I didn't wear the brace at Salute," Johnson said.

Johnson was able to practice that Saturday, as was Shekinna Stricklen. "Awesome," Assistant Coach Mickie DeMoss said about having the pair on the practice court. "It's hard to win games without those two. I was very pleased, especially with Stricklen, because I didn't know what to expect from her coming off that injury. But she moved pretty well . . . and hopefully by Monday she'll be full speed." Tennessee had not yet been at full strength this season with the entire slate of 11 players. When junior guard Kamiko Williams was activated in late December, Spani was sidelined. The coaches would relish having a full roster, even a rather beat-up one. "It just gives you more choices as a coach," DeMoss said. "Also, it helps the competition amongst your team. They know they've got to compete for minutes, and you hope that intensifies their play." Johnson would be in the lineup; sore shoulder and all, she didn't miss a game all season. "Tylenol, play through it," she said. "Forget about the pain. I will be on the floor."

Although All-American guard Skylar Diggins got the lion's share of the media attention, DeMoss said Notre Dame presented a team-wide challenge. "If in one word I could describe Notre Dame it's tough," DeMoss said. She handled the scouting report for the Tennessee-Notre Dame game and was asked what the Irish liked to do on offense. "Score," DeMoss deadpanned. "In every way imaginable." She really wasn't kidding. "They are putting up a lot of points," DeMoss said. "They like points off their defense, they lead the nation in steals, they like to push in transition, and their half-court execution is some of the best that I've seen from any team in the country as far as their pure execution. Vanderbilt is always a great team in our league that executes well, and they're a Vanderbilt with better players."

The game would be a homecoming of sorts for Briana Bass, but a week-night game with a late tip at a venue 150 miles away from her hometown of Indianapolis would limit her family presence at the game. However, Tim and Gina Bass, the parents of the senior guard, made the trip to the northern area of the state, despite the significant snowfall in the area. Bass had earned the respect and admiration of her teammates for being willing to play a role for the team off the bench. She also was one of the hardest

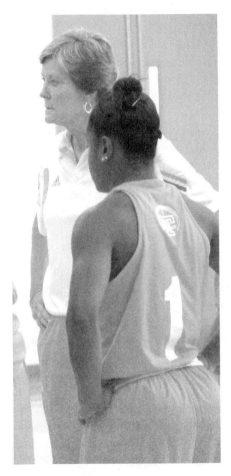

Briana Bass with Pat Summitt at practice. Bass would erupt in tears after the final loss and thank Summitt for making her the woman she became in college.

workers in practice despite getting limited game minutes. "We've needed her in a lot of situations," Manning said. "I am just very proud of her for sticking with it."

Bass did stick with Tennessee and her senior class. "My family and God and my teammates have really kept me focused," said Bass, whose tearful thanks to Pat Summitt at the end of the season for making "me the woman I am today" would become part of an ESPN documentary about the head coach. "I wanted to stay and play hard for them. My family has taught me to never give up on my dreams, and my dream was to play basketball." Bass' ability to go home and see her parents was one of the few bright spots of the game. And while the Irish players and staff didn't wear anything related to "We Back Pat"—the only time that happened on the road during the 2011–12 season—the Notre Dame fans shouted support to Summitt and gave her a rousing ovation.

Other than that, Tennessee likely wanted to burn the game tape. "I just want to apologize to the fans. We just were not very good, and we were not in Notre Dame's league. We didn't compete," Holly Warlick said after the game. "We knew it was going to be a great game when we walked out and saw a sea of green," McGraw said. "It was an awesome sight. I think it really fired the team up and got us so engaged." When one coach opened her press conference with an apology and the other noted the T-shirt color of the fans, it was a good indicator of how the game went. Tennessee was steamrolled before a sold-out crowd of 9,149 at Purcell Pavilion at the Joyce Center.

Taber Spani was released on game day. It didn't help against the Irish—a very rusty Spani was 0–2 in nine minutes of play and she missed the next practice—and the Lady Vols got little offense from anywhere else on the court. They set a program record for fewest points scored in a game and were buried 72–44. Notre Dame found its offensive rhythm, shooting 67.9 percent in the second half and pouring in 44 points after leading 28–18 at halftime. The Fighting Irish were clearly peeved—they were bringing full court pressure with two minutes left in the game, and Diggins remained in the game until the final 67 seconds. "It's not their job to keep the game close. It was shaking the bully off of their back in front of their home fans," said Dean Lockwood, referring to the series having been so lopsided in Tennessee's favor. "They have high respect for Pat."

Indeed, in 2014 when the Final Four was being played in Nashville, and one storyline was the escalating bitterness between Notre Dame and Connecticut, McGraw had this to say about Summitt: "I think all women's coaches really respect her and looked up to her, because they knew when she spoke, it was about what was good for the women's game. She role-modeled how to be gracious in victory, as well as defeat. She was such a classy coach and, unfortunately, the game and sportsmanship lost a lot when we lost her." Summitt was on her feet quite a bit during the game, but the players could not sustain any energy. "I remembered how distraught I was," Lockwood said. "I think in the final six or seven minutes, our kids kind of quit. We felt like this is insurmountable. They went from 100 to 80 to 60 really fast. It was really disappointing."

Assistant coaches are often on the road during the season, whether traveling for away games or crisscrossing the country to recruit. It is not unusual for them to join the team on the road from a recruiting trip. The job means a lot of time alone, from plane flights to rented cars to hotel stays. Coaches tend to stay in the moment, and Tennessee's assistants were especially focused on what was directly in front of them during the 2011–12 season: next practice, next film session, next game. But Lockwood specifically remembers a drive to Indianapolis for a recruiting trip during which his mind was on Summitt.

"There were some times behind the wheel of a car where I thought about it, and I thought about Pat and her life, how special it was to work with her. You're alone in your car. You've got a long plane flight. You're by yourself. You're not with the team. So there were moments those thoughts were definitely there. Rather than break down, the words I would use is there would be periodic moments of sadness where you feel sad, not pity, but sadness because of someone so great and someone of such impact and such incredible depth of character and substance and such positive mentoring to anybody that she encounters, that it was slowly waning. It was a slow leak. It's not going to ever be full again."

19

SEASON OF ADJUSTMENT

Holly Warlick took on a tremendous amount of responsibility that season. Assistant coaches do a lot behind the scenes, from days and nights on the road for recruiting to the preparation of scouting reports that take hours of film breakdown, followed by detailed written summaries of plays and personnel to present to the team at practice and in the film room. Warlick retained all of those duties while also serving in what essentially amounted to a co-head coach position as the season progressed. "I admire the entire coaching staff and the entire support staff for what they did that year for Holly and for Pat," Jenny Moshak said. "Holly rose to the occasion. There is no doubt about it. In other situations you might have had egos take over and that was not the case. Now, was there stumbling along the way? Absolutely. We all stumbled."

The season was unprecedented in sports. Coaches have continued amid family crisis, health concerns, and team tragedy. No coach had ever announced dementia and then proceeded to stay in the public eye. It took tremendous courage on the part of Summitt and perseverance on the part

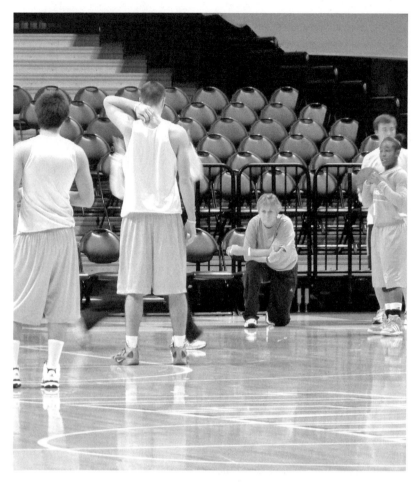

Holly Warlick watches practice during the final season. Warlick and the other assistants adjusted daily, depending on what Pat Summitt needed in terms of on-court help.

of the players. "It made us work harder I think," Vicki Baugh said. "It really brought us together. We looked at it like something that won't affect this woman. We were thinking she is strong enough to get by. The first thing I was happy to hear was that she is still going to be part of the team and she is still going to be coaching. That is what I was concerned about. It made us feel closer. It made me work harder in rehab and get myself together. Everything I had been through, I realized this is nothing."

Baugh was a fifth-year senior, already wise beyond her years. Meighan Simmons was a sophomore reeling from the news that a woman she had worshipped from afar before arriving in Knoxville was stricken by a disease. Simmons was a freshman in the 2010–11 season. "I didn't think anything was wrong. Honestly, I felt I got the full Pat, that full effect. I did notice she stopped yelling at me. I don't know if she was getting comfortable with me because of the position I was in or because of that. It could be both." Simmons was thrust into the point guard spot despite having never played the position, even in high school. Summitt was inclined to go easier on the first-year player under those circumstances—she loved Simmons' aggressive nature on offense and didn't want to squelch it—but the absence of yelling was unusual. Of course, Simmons, a late recruit for Tennessee after a scholarship became available for medical reasons, didn't have the historical context to realize that was an aberration.

Simmons definitely saw some differences as a sophomore. "Her tone of voice was different. She wasn't raising her voice. Her aura was so much more mellow and relaxed. She was subdued at times. If Pat was having trouble getting her point across or expressing her frustration, Holly expressed it. It was like, 'I'm mom, you're daughter; you do what I say because I am telling you what to do.' Pat was expressing her feelings through Holly. It was very different. Seeing her in a different light and having to understand where she was and what she was going through, it motivated me to work 10 times harder and not take anything for granted. But emotionally it wore on me to the point in practice where I would be like, 'Oh, man.'"

Simmons idolized Summitt, who became a second mother to her during her freshman year. While things changed on the court, the maternal connection with Summitt continued during Simmons' sophomore season. "It was a mother-daughter bond. She created this motherly aura with the players that she'd had before me. And I took advantage of that. I am not saying she compares to my mom but a surrogate mother. When I saw her she would say, 'Are you eating well? Are you doing well in classes?' She just made sure that my well-being was OK. That kept me continuing to come back to her. I wanted her to know I still had that relationship with her. I was still able to communicate with her and make her feel like she was still a part of me because I so wanted her to feel that."

Baugh approached the situation as if nothing had changed. "I stayed the same. I tried to treat her the same no matter what. We talked to Tyler about it and he was like, 'Just stay the same with her.' And knowing how Pat is, she wouldn't want anyone to feel sorry for her and treat her any differently.

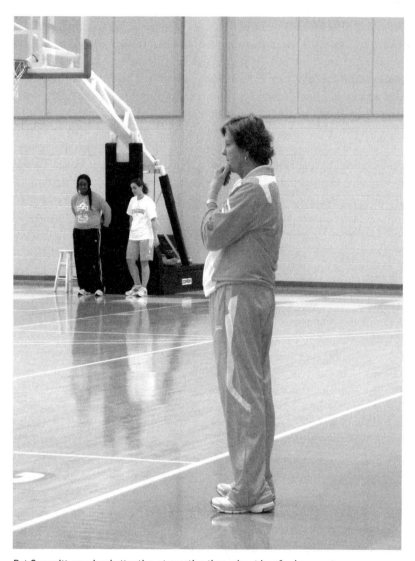

Pat Summitt remained attentive at practice throughout her final season.

Even if she was having an off day, I would still ask her the same questions. I would go to her with any situations. We did our best to not let it affect how we would normally treat her. If something wasn't answered or we could see this is not one of her best days, we would go to the other coaches. She was still involved in the practices, and she was still yelling at us."

Tyler Summitt was the one to accompany his mother to the Mayo Clinic, where the illness was discovered and confirmed in late May 2011. One of Pat's closest friends, Mary Margaret Carter—a Chi Omega sorority sister when both were at Tennessee-Martin and a surgical nurse—also made the trip. The news was devastating.

"We went to the beach shortly after the diagnosis, and that was a good time to be away from everything and come to grips with things," Tyler said. "Mom decided she wanted to go public and decided that she wanted to keep coaching. And that is what we ended up doing. We had to get everybody on the same page because of what it meant for her team and her program."

When Pat Summitt met with Chancellor Jimmy Cheek and then-acting Athletics Director Joan Cronan, they told her she could coach at Tennessee until she was ready to step aside. (Cronan would step aside shortly after that meeting when Dave Hart was hired as athletics director.) The next step was to tell the players. Tyler was at that team meeting. "I definitely respect all those players for how they handled everything and also for embracing my mom. They really loved her and surrounded her and supported her. I think they also realized that she was still teaching them another lesson to not be scared of life's circumstances and to not let things affect your work ethic and to focus on what you can control. Mom said, 'Listen, this is not going to be a pity party. We are going to focus on our team.' That set the tone for the year."

"Business as usual" became the theme as Summitt and her staff wanted to keep things as normal as possible for the players while also accepting that matters had irrevocably changed. "As a staff, there wasn't a blueprint on how to deal with it, so we just had to try to manage it and make sure Pat was taken care of the best way we could," Mickie DeMoss said. "When you're in the throes of it, and it's a day-to-day thing. . . . Was it difficult? Absolutely it was difficult. It still is. But we managed. We got through it. Pat did a great job." Summitt's willingness to be the working face of the disease with national scrutiny was unprecedented. It was even more remarkable considering how Summitt had been able to juggle so much at one time. There were epic stories about her laser focus, including the oft-told tale of her coming home one evening still in basketball mode and not noticing a new car parked in her garage. Now, she was willing to let the world watch her adjust.

"I think Pat's transparency helped, because I know how strong-willed she is, and before any of this happened and before she went public with it, she could have a hundred things going wrong that day, but she would never let anyone know," Taber Spani said. "She also embraced her role of becoming more of an off-the-court coach for the kids and understanding that, yes, Holly had to do more of the head coach duties, per se, of the film work and the Xs and Os. In the huddle, she would start joking. Stuff you would never hear Pat do before. She embraced that role of becoming a friend to the team and being there for them. She became really personable. For the girls who hadn't built that relationship before, they really got to know her in a way they might not have known her."

Spani already had that kind of relationship with Summitt. So did Baugh. But they both also knew that some days Summitt would not be able to take that role. The staff was always candid with the media that season, reminding them that Summitt would have good days and bad ones. That was the reality of dementia. "I always go to Pat about everything," Baugh said. "I had Dean, but he's a man, so he doesn't always understand every time. So when I

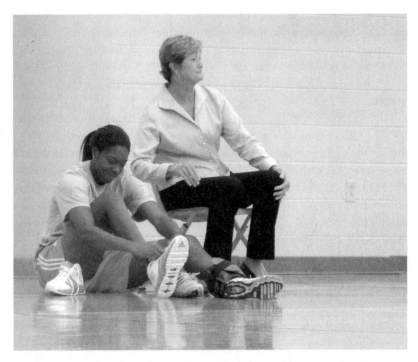

Pat Summitt, who had been at a speaking engagement, shares a pre-practice conversation in 2009 with Vicki Baugh. The two became very close, as Summitt was a surrogate mother to Baugh.

needed to talk to my 'mom' at Tennessee, that part was kind of rough. I had to grow closer to a lot of my teammates." Detailed instructions came from the assistant coaches. The players had to adjust to tuning in to a different voice, especially in practice.

If Simmons got tired in workouts, she had a ready-made cure for fatigue: "Think about Pat," Simmons said. "It created this aura of dedication and passion and hard work. I had that hunger, but that just brought extra fire. My flame has not gone out, and it's because of her that I still have that flame." Warlick also kept a frenetic pace all season. She profusely perspired during some games, though Summitt's sense of humor prevailed there, too, as she would ask her former player why she had to sweat so much. "I was doing a little bit of everything and that's OK. You run on adrenaline. You run with the understanding that you're trying to keep what Pat built," Warlick said.

Moshak, meanwhile, kept a close eye on Summitt for obvious reasons. "When you are in pain with Alzheimer's the pain fibers take over and you can't cognitively process because the pain moves so quickly through the neurological system," Moshak said. "So if we can minimize the pain, that gives us a better chance with the thought process and she can work on game plans and watch film." Moshak watched Summitt for such signs as increased limping, and she scheduled more treatment and made sure Summitt got ice packs. Summitt eventually had knee and ankle surgeries after retirement, which tremendously lessened her pain.

Of course, Moshak also tried to keep an eye on Warlick. "I think she did extremely well and under fire, which obviously was seen by the administration in hiring her for the position," Moshak said. "But it doesn't mean it wasn't a challenge and emotionally draining to her as well. Holly had to sacrifice a lot that season in terms of self-care to take care of all these other things, including her mentor." Still, Moshak's primary responsibility was to the student-athletes, and her process that last season was to make sure she delivered the injury report to Warlick as well as Summitt.

The toughest adjustment for Warlick was watching the woman she had known for decades—Warlick began playing for Summitt in 1976—have to change how she coached. While Summitt still talked to the team before, during, and after games, the assistants handled a lot of in-game tasks, including calling plays and setting the defense. Substitutions were done by committee, and Summitt continued her input there. "That probably was the hardest thing for me, seeing her move away from leading the team," Warlick said. "One thing about Pat is she has given me a lot of responsibility before all of this happened so it helped me."

Baugh had seen Summitt at her best during the successful quest for a national title in 2008. In her final year, Baugh saw a scaled-back Summitt. "Hearing her voice in practice, hearing her running off our plays, the impact she had on our coaches, all of that made a difference," Baugh said. "Not getting that stare . . . you need that drive to play. It was very difficult. It is hard to watch someone you love go through that." But Summitt could still deliver the thunder when needed. She may have accepted a reduced role as far as daily tasks were concerned, but she still commanded considerable presence. "She still had a clear vision: 'We're not boxing out, we're not rebounding, we're not pushing the ball, we're not getting back,'" Warlick said.

Television cameras seemed determined to stay on Summitt if she in any way looked as if she were not occupied with the game. It was an inherently unfair and inaccurate portrayal of the coach. Newspaper and wire service photographers shot multiple photos of Summitt throughout the game, and their galleries offered a much-needed portrayal of her. She was shown talking to players—Cierra Burdick got an earful from Summitt in Athens against Georgia—standing up and directing traffic, and talking to officials. The corporation that is Lady Vols basketball went smoothly, a credit to the system Summitt had built and maintained for decades. "We had been doing it so long that it just flowed; it just happened. We got it done," Warlick said. "But the day-to-day practice, the game prep, that was tough. And I was very sensitive and aware that people were asking, 'What's wrong with Pat?' And I didn't like that."

DeMoss had been with the Lady Vols for nearly two decades and then returned after an absence of eight years. It was a seamless transition. "When you're a great leader, as Pat is, the program almost was running itself," DeMoss said. "It wasn't as difficult as if you were taking over for someone who did not have a strong grip on the program, who did not have her philosophy in place and didn't have good players on the team. It wasn't as emotionally demanding as what was going on with Pat and trying to intertwine that all together. I think just having the mental ability and toughness to compartmentalize and be able to deal with what you had to deal with on the court and help Pat and navigate that whole situation, you had to be really focused and pay attention to detail and make sure that everything went as smoothly for her as possible." Tyler was present as often as he could be while balancing being an honor student and basketball player, and he made it a point to point out what the staff did for his mother. "The amount that Holly, Mickie and Dean stepped up that year was absolutely incredible," Tyler said. "They did a lot of extra work so Mom could focus on her health."

For coaches and players the 94-foot-by-50-foot court and its sidelines should become a sanctuary. That was no longer the case.

Cierra Burdick was just a freshman that season. She acknowledged that the stress of the situation took its toll at times on the players. "It was like we had three head coaches almost. That got difficult at times. We didn't necessarily know who to look to at times and when to look to them. That was tough on the players as well as the coaches. It kind of took away our ability to focus on ball."

The impact that Summitt had on her players can't be overstated. To see a woman who was the embodiment of strength compromised in any way by an insidious disease made them feel as if their own hearts were under siege. "I think the most difficult part of it is Pat is the strongest woman that I have ever met. Just hearing her . . . the way she told us she didn't want any pity or anyone to feel sorry for her. She made it almost to where we can fight this out together," Baugh said. "Initially, I would have been so sad but I was like, 'She can overcome this. She is just so strong of a person, I thought this couldn't hold her down.' Unfortunately, the kind of the disease it is, I am just now realizing what kind of impact this really has. Even the strongest person I have ever met, it has an effect on them, too."

Moshak was as attuned to the players' minds as she was to ensuring they were physically able to play basketball. Since she spent so much time in the role of caregiver, the players would talk to her about anything. "To be honest the country, the university, Knoxville, Tennessee, have no clue what that team had to endure that year," Moshak said. "It was unbelievably emotionally challenging on so many levels. Some of them felt like they had been ripped off because they were recruited by her and they wanted four years with her. Some feeling extremely motivated and trying to do it all. Some questioning faith as to why. They are trying to balance school, their relationships, playing basketball, supporting a coach.

"I admire that team for what they accomplished under the consistent stress emotionally, spiritually, mentally, and even physically, because that emotional stuff drains you physically and to be able to perform and set yourself aside when you're in pain and try to go out and succeed is extremely tiresome and extremely honorable and admirable. I was so proud of that team for the strength that they had through that process. To ask that of 18 to 22 year olds is really tough. And they're still dealing with school, stuff from home, all the issues from college and then navigating the press and the fans all asking questions. They were constantly reminded. Just navigating through a storm, and it is a storm we knew was coming, but you're still in the storm."

20

SEC BATTLES

The best thing for Tennessee after the disappointment at Notre Dame was to return to SEC play with road trips to close out the month of January. They would head to Tuscaloosa to play Alabama and then Athens for a rematch with Georgia.

The Lady Vol coaches discussed the starting lineup right up until game time at Foster Auditorium on the campus of the Crimson Tide and opted to give freshman Cierra Burdick her first career nod and senior Briana Bass her first of the season. Burdick had reached out to Pat Summitt earlier in the season to ask about playing time—like any competitor, she wanted more of it. "I remember sitting down with her and discussing playing time," Burdick said. "And she was like, 'You've got to earn that.' She would tell me to be patient. Your time is coming. It's a process, and you've got to continue to grow and learn."

The five starters set the tone from the opening tip when Glory Johnson found Bass for a three-pointer, much to the delight of the Lady Vols bench. "I was really proud that we came out the way we did," said Summitt, who posed for photos and signed autographs for Lady Vol and Crimson Tide fans on the court after the game while waiting for her players to get ready to depart. "Across the board, this is a feel-good game. Everybody got to play, everybody played significant minutes and made a difference."

"When I talked to Briana Bass, I said, 'Let's go,'" said Glory Johnson, who always advocated for Bass. After Bass' trey ball, Johnson and Vicki Baugh rattled off 13 points between them and the Lady Vols led by double digits less than six minutes into the game. Those wearing orange among the 2,049 in the stands—and there were quite a few scattered throughout the auditorium—enjoyed the start of the game. The result of a lineup under the reward plan was an 86–56 romp over Alabama, allowing Tennessee to shake off some of the stench from the defeat at Notre Dame.

The players were also likely happy to be in a game that Thursday evening. It had to be less demanding than the practice they endured Wednesday because they at least got breaks on the bench in Tuscaloosa. "We killed them on Wednesday," Holly Warlick said, referring to what may have been the toughest practice of the season, which is unheard of the day before a game. But it speaks to the profound disappointment after getting destroyed by the Irish in South Bend, a loss Warlick said was the biggest letdown since Ball State bounced the Lady Vols out of the first round of the NCAA tourney in 2009.

Warlick opened her press conference in Indiana with an apology for how the Lady Vols played. In Alabama three days later, she was laughing at the responses of Kamiko Williams, who was still working her way into basketball shape after knee rehab. She played in both halves and entered with 10:59 left to play after Meighan Simmons had to leave with a bloodied nose. Williams' goal had been to log hard, sustained effort in two-minute segments. When she saw Burdick at the scorer's table at the 8:53 mark, she pointed at her chest but Burdick pointed to a teammate. Williams said she had hoped the relief was her. "I am not going to lie, Coach," Williams said to laughter from Warlick.

"A lot of times she wants out, and I just ignore her," Warlick joked.

When Shekinna Stricklen went down after a collision under the basket with an Alabama player and had to leave with 8:20 to play, Simmons, whose nose was now OK, took her place. That meant Williams had to stay on the court. She ended up finishing the game and logged 11 consecutive minutes. Next up for Tennessee was the third consecutive road game of the week with a trip to Athens. Georgia can be an enigmatic team, and also one that typically plays so much better at home at Stegeman Coliseum.

Despite being freshmen that season, Burdick and Ariel Massengale logged a lot of minutes. They often had media interview duties, too, because both were key players, and they both handled the media well. When Burdick walked onto the court for a scheduled interview, Massengale was still finishing up her media session. Burdick grabbed a basketball and headed to the other end of the arena to get up some shots while she waited. That epitomized the first-year forward from Charlotte, North Carolina. Her offensive efficiency and willingness to work led to additional playing time. Summitt had lamented at times that season that she had to constantly remind players to get up extra shots on their own to maintain offensive consistency, but Burdick wasn't on the reminder list. Despite a full course load in the classroom and mandatory study hall for freshmen, Burdick was a regular in the gym outside of practice. "I am a gym rat, so it's no problem for me," Burdick said. "I get my studying hours in and I get my food in and I get my school in. If I have to come in here at 10 o'clock at night then I am in here at 10 o'clock at night just getting shots up."

It had only been three weeks since the two teams had last played, but Burdick said she would need a refresher on the game and scouting report. "So much stuff has happened between Georgia games," Burdick said. Tennessee wanted to maintain its league momentum. Georgia wanted redemption. "I think about the game up there, which easily qualifies as our poorest performance of the year," Coach Andy Landers said. "Our players know that. They understand what didn't happen that needed to happen. I think you'll see a very energized, enthused and excited basketball team trying to make amends for the game in Knoxville."

That Sunday afternoon, a sold-out crowd of 10,523 (including Andraya Carter, a high school senior who had signed with Tennessee) greeted the Lady Vols, and while Lady Bulldog fans were the majority, orange-clad fans were clustered throughout the arena and made their voices heard throughout the game. It was hard to tell what the Lady Vols were happier about after the game—the win over rival Georgia or the fact that they were headed home. After leading by just one point at the break, Tennessee claimed a 67–50 victory.

Taber Spani returned for Tennessee, and her presence on the court changed the opponent's defensive strategy. The impact of her absence became readily apparent in the month of January. The most impressive number in the box score for Spani was the number of minutes played at 21. Spani swished her first three, and that changed the way Georgia guarded Tennessee. It came right after Massengale drained a three-pointer, and with two shooters to track, the Lady Bulldogs increased the perimeter pressure. That opened up driving lanes, and Shekinna Stricklen took advantage, especially in the second half. She got to the rim and led all scorers with 24 points.

Spani's defender would not leave her, because Spani's step-back three meant the defense had to stay close. Stricklen took full advantage and headed to the rim. "That's the best part about it," Stricklen said. "You go to her side and if you just beat your man, you've got a wide-open layup, because people are not going to help off of her." The Lady Vols opened February with two home games against South Carolina and Auburn. The players, who had missed several classes with so much travel, were happy to be in Knoxville. So were the coaches. "It's absolutely wonderful," said Mickie DeMoss, who used a day at home to get her cast removed and replace it with a brace for her right arm.

Spani was happy to finally be back on the court after a frustrating rehab that required a lot of rest. While she was not 100 percent yet—Pat Summitt noted a little Spani goes a long way—she had at least returned to practice. "As a competitor, the hardest thing to do is to sit out," Spani said. "It's a joy to be on the floor." She sustained the bone bruise Nov. 20, 2011, after being knocked to the floor by a Virginia player celebrating a made basket and a foul for what is called an "and-one" play since the shooter also gets to take a free throw. Spani never saw the collision coming, and she got hit in the knee and then slammed the knee on the court.

Opponents defend Spani as if every shot could go in, so just her presence on the court helped teammates. Massengale realized it against Georgia on one possession and drove to the basket. She faked a pass to Spani, whose defender stayed put instead of rotating to help on Massengale, and she had a clear path to the rim. "The girl stayed on me, and she got a wide-open layup, because they've got to respect shooters in the corners," Spani said. Summitt had concerns about the next opponent. She continued to watch film, and South Carolina had her attention. "If you had to vote at this point of the season, the most improved team would have to be South Carolina," Summitt said of the SEC. "They're athletic and they score the ball well. We're going to have our hands full."

Those words would turn out to be prophetic. The Lady Vols suffered their first defeat at home in SEC play in 28 games after South Carolina took down Tennessee 64–60. The busload of South Carolina fans among the 15,021 in attendance at Thompson-Boling Arena on February 2 made themselves heard at the end of the game with a "USC" chant as the celebration began in front of the Gamecocks bench. South Carolina defeated

Tennessee for the first time since 1980, and the Lady Vols had sustained their first defeat at home in the SEC in four years. LSU had been the last league team to claim a win in Knoxville in 2008. "To say we didn't play particularly well for 40 minutes tonight would be an understatement, but you have to credit South Carolina for that," Summitt said. "They executed a great game plan from start to finish and showed it over and over and over for 40 minutes."

The Gamecocks took a page out of Summitt's book and won the game with offensive rebounding, none bigger than the one at the end of the game that allowed South Carolina to seal the win at the free throw line and keep the ball away from Tennessee. Johnson, who became a team leader that season, offered no excuses for the poor performance after the game. "We have the fan support," Johnson said. "We have home-court advantage. We're sleeping in our own beds before the game. We're having a great pregame meal. We're completely prepared with the scouting report from our coaches, so this loss is on us. I can't think of one thing that I could give you as an excuse for why we lost this game, but we just weren't ready to play. Our defense was awful."

South Carolina Coach Dawn Staley and her team presented Tyler Summitt with a check for $20,000 for the Alzheimer's Association in honor of his mother that they raised via donations and pledges after the team participated in a fundraiser walk before the season. Tennessee native and South Carolina football Coach Steve Spurrier, who was in attendance and was a close friend of Summitt's, made a major contribution. "She just said great job," Staley said when asked what Summitt said after the game. "She did come up to us before the game and thanked us for backing her. It is truly our pleasure, and I'm glad our players got a chance to have this experience, knowing the tradition of Tennessee, and by far, this is the biggest win of my career."

Johnson was still seething, and her mood didn't improve much until the next day at practice. She called out the team as a whole in the post-game press conference, especially for their lack of attention to the defensive scouting report. "It took me not sleeping and talking about it with my teammates and I just let it all out that night and kind of got over it," said Johnson, who also stewed over her missed layup late in the game. "I talked to a lot of the seniors. This is our last chance. We have to go to work. Everyone has to pick up their game, including myself."

By February, the fuel in the regular season tank is starting to run low. Players are banged up after a month in the SEC, the most physical and deepest conference, top to bottom, in the country. The last-place team can give the first-place one a close game and even pull off the upset. That essentially doesn't happen in other women's basketball conferences. Add to that mix the fact the Lady Vols were in the midst of a season in which their head coach was dealing with early onset dementia, and it's easy to understand why they would stumble. Summitt modified her style to lessen stress to her body and mind and allowed her assistants to handle a lot of the in-game shouting to players who were used to responding to Summitt's voice.

The senior class had been through an unprecedented series of events. It began with a loss in the first round of the NCAA Tournament in 2009—the Lady Vols had always reached at least the Sweet 16 since the tourney began in 1982—and then the personal traumas began. Midway through the 2008–09 season, Baugh again tore the ACL in her left knee and entered another grueling rehab process. Teammate Amber Gray suffered a stroke from a brain aneurysm and nearly died in July 2009. In October 2009, Assistant Coach Daedra Charles Furlow, a former Lady Vol whose jersey has been retired, told the team she had breast cancer. During the seniors' time on campus, they had watched three teammates have their Division I careers ended prematurely by injury—point guards Cait McMahan and Lauren Avant and center Kelley Cain. Former Lady Vol Melissa McCray, who lived in Knoxville, spoke to the team in 2009 about having a fighting spirit as she battled breast cancer. She died December 27, 2010, and the players wore No. 35 commemorative patches for the remainder of that season.

They witnessed tragedy on and off the court, and they also saw people prevail. Gray restarted her career at Xavier, where she was closer to her hometown doctors. Charles-Furlow survived, served as the team's director of character development, and coached high school basketball. McMahan is a successful recording artist with performances on ESPN's College Game-Day. Avant transferred to Rhodes College, underwent additional surgery, resurrected her basketball career at the Division III level, and went into coaching. Cain's chronic pain in her knees and hip ebbed with a year off the court, and she became a professional basketball player.

Baugh's sense of perspective was expected for a fifth-year senior, but freshman Isabelle Harrison, who has 11 siblings, also understood that sometimes life can stagger a person. The native of Nashville was about 11 years old when that lesson hit home. "Having Pat diagnosed it reminded me of when my brother got diagnosed with lupus, and my mom had to give one of her kidneys for him to live," Harrison said. "I remember her being in the hospital and him doing dialysis. I remember how hard it was, but we were there for each other and people were helping us out, too. Just like with Pat, people are coming for her every game. When you have people support you, it helps. My brother is still living, and Pat was still our coach."

That senior class, through all of its ups and downs, consistently responded to one thing: the sheer force of Summitt's will and her ability to snap a player to attention. "I do," Johnson said with a smile when asked if she missed Summitt yelling at her. "It's something that we do miss. And she's still there. Don't get me wrong. It still happens, just not as often. We know that there are certain things that we are doing wrong, and we try to hold each other accountable, but it's not the same thing if Pat is holding you accountable. When Pat says it, that's the end of the story. That's it. If she says it, you've got to do it."

Auburn provided the necessary court tonic. The 82–61 win over the Tigers pleased the head coach. The Lady Vols did it by getting the ball inside and ratcheting up the defense. "Three stats jump off the page . . . our points in the paint (52–28 in Tennessee's favor) and our points off of turnovers (21–2)," Summitt said. "Those are on the positive side. On the negative side, I don't like the fact that we were outrebounded by Auburn (42–39)." Midway through the first half, Summitt inserted Kamiko Williams and handled several substitutions during the game. "Pat is Pat," Warlick said. "I'll say this: She still gets up and has a voice when we need to make a point, and that's what I love about her. She gets in the huddle, and she gets on them pretty heavily. She may pick and choose when she does, but when she does, it's pretty powerful."

Some power was delivered in a small package, too, when Briana Bass entered the game to bring some defensive pressure against Auburn's point guard, Najat Ouardad. Bass brought the crowd of 16,361 to its feet when she stole the ball out of a trap near the scorer's table and passed ahead to Shekinna Stricklen while falling out of bounds. Bass also stole an in-bounds pass near Auburn's bench and found Taber Spani for the layup, which caused the crowd to erupt again. "Bree is feisty and her teammates love her energy and feed off of it," Summitt said. "She plays with a great deal of heart."

Usually, the 5'2" Bass would be the tiniest one on the court, but her Auburn counterpart was the 5'1" Ouardad. "Bree finally found somebody she's taller than today," Warlick said afterwards. As Bass smothered Auburn's ball handler, the fans roared their approval, and the energy filtered to the rest of the team. "As soon as she came in, not only did the crowd go crazy, but our energy level picked up, and we were playing high-pressure defense," Spani said. "Bree was the point person on that, and we love it for her, and she's had such a great attitude throughout everything."

"Everything" could mean quite a lot for this team that season: it had already taken on six regular season losses—Tennessee was 17–6 at that point with two SEC losses—due in part to the fact that its iconic head coach had to adjust her daily role. But when Stricklen, whose play of late had been shaky on both ends, wanted to address the slippage in her game, she sought Summitt. "Shekinna came to me and asked to visit," Summitt said. "I told her how much we counted on her as our All-American to work hard and bring it every day and to set an example for her teammates. I told her we needed her to step up and play the way she is capable of playing."

The conversation was effective because Stricklen played with high energy on both ends of the floor in the first game after that conversation. Of the senior class as a whole, Stricklen, who has acknowledged how laid-back she can be, was the one player who needed Summitt to dial her up at times. It was a big step for Stricklen to seek out Summitt, rather than the other way around, as the laconic senior was likely to keep to herself. "It just feels good when I hear her voice. It really does get to me. Just listening to what she was telling me was great," Stricklen said. "We really needed to talk."

But the SEC is a two-month battle that wears down every team in the league. It can also get a bit batty. The Lady Vols had two rematches on tap: a trip to Nashville against Vanderbilt and the arrival of Kentucky in Knoxville. The Lady Vols dissected Vanderbilt earlier in the season, but games at Memorial Gymnasium with its bizarre configuration could get interesting. The Commodores also put considerable effort into keeping Lady Vols out of the lower level. Orange-clad fans usually found the only ticket availability in the upper reaches with empty seats below them.

Lady Vol players subbing in to the game needed to remember to turn right, because the Tennessee bench was on one baseline, but habits are hard to break: players are used to going past the coaches on the way to the scorer's table. At Memorial Gymnasium, they head away from the Lady Vol coaches, whose seats are closer to the basket support. It would be the first time Ariel Massengale played in the bastardized gym, and it can be a challenge for any first-year player—especially the point guard. With the benches on the baseline, the players often have their backs to their coaches, and they can't hear them 94 feet away.

Of greater concern for the Lady Vols before that game was their team defense. Since the heady days of back-to-back national titles in 2007 and 2008, the Lady Vols had struggled defensively, specifically too often allowing one player on the opposing team to erupt. Those players were often perimeter ones, though Stanford forward Nneka Ogwumike was a notable exception. Johnson was the player most capable of stopping an onslaught on the perimeter, but the coaches had to weigh what they lost elsewhere on the court, namely post defense and boards from the 6–3 forward if she had to guard a player away from the basket. They were also aware of foul trouble becoming an issue. The loss to South Carolina was partly attributable to Johnson being parked on the bench because of whistles.

It was a role that Nicky Anosike had embraced. Anosike was a post player who wanted to guard whoever was scoring against the Lady Vols. "Nicky was one of those who, 'OK, where are we getting hurt? Let me be the one.' She would be the one that would go charge the machine gun nest," Dean Lockwood said. "That is Nicky: 'If we're taking fire, who's doing it? And if no one else is taking them out, I'll be the one and take a couple of volunteers.'"

It was also a role that Johnson was ready to accept if she got turned loose. "She's become more and more of that," Lockwood said of Johnson during her senior year. Johnson also had the physical skills to match the desire. "As far as the combination of strength, speed, explosion and stamina, you rarely get that (in one player)," Anosike had the muscle and staying power, but Johnson had sprinter's speed and a high jumper's hops, too.

"She's got a first and second step that she can cut you off. She's cat-like in quickness, and she also has got straight-away speed. That combination is a very gifted athlete and a very imposing defender," Lockwood said. If (the archangel) Gabriel sat down and said, 'We're going to draw up a prototype body for a defensive player,' right there, Glory Johnson."

Tennessee needed a team full of those players for the game against Vanderbilt. The game didn't tip until 9 p.m. Eastern (8 p.m. in Nashville) on a Thursday, so the players had all day and into the evening to wait with an overnight bus ride back to Knoxville so they could be in class Friday morning. To make matters worse, Summitt was violently ill with a stomach virus. She was dehydrated from the ordeal and had barely slept. She likely should have stayed at the hotel, but she knew if she weren't on the sideline, the media would focus on her dementia and blame the disease for her absence. So while she made it to Memorial Gymnasium, Summitt likely wished she had never seen the game.

The game in Nashville between the in-state rivals is often attended by the capital's political figures, and Governor Bill Haslam was present and sitting behind Tennessee's bench, along with Summitt's family. Summitt's demeanor during the game was concerning, but Knoxville and Nashville newspaper writers and columnists learned in the media room before the game that Summitt was ill. That didn't stop a columnist for *The Tennessean* from writing a piece with a headline that stated: "Pat Summitt loses her grip on the Lady Vols." While no one would deny that dementia had an effect on Summitt, the column went too far too soon and equated her sideline demeanor with the disease, as if she were too addled to even know what was happening. Summitt was understandably livid when she read it. It was a narrative she could ill afford that season.

The headline across the *InsideTennessee* story after the game was: "Lady Vols scorched by Vandy." They entered the game in the thick of the conference race and stumbled badly with a 93–79 loss. The Commodores had four players tally double figures, and Jasmine Lister reached a double-double with 19 points and 13 assists. Tiffany Clarke got one, too, in traditional fashion with 23 points and 12 rebounds. Tennessee was shredded at the rim with Vanderbilt getting 52 points in the paints compared to just 28 for the Lady Vols. "We weren't communicating, hands weren't high, we weren't contesting shots," Johnson said. "A lot of wide open three-pointers that went in, and there was no one around. At a game like this, you've got to forget about the offense and focus on playing defense."

Tennessee managed to wipe out a 10-point deficit in the second half with a collection of starters and bench players. The Lady Vols scored 45 points after the break, but Vanderbilt, which added 51 points after halftime, continued to get the shots it wanted out of its offense with the bulk of them coming close to the rim. "Obviously, we are very disappointed and rightfully so," Summitt said. "We saw a lot of lack of effort on the court. You have to give Vanderbilt all the credit. They came ready to play. Melanie Balcomb does a great job." Balcomb thanked the students for creating a true home court advantage—Tennessee fans were definitely present, though they were not the majority among the crowd of 12,034—and said if the students did that every game, the Commodores would be undefeated at home.

Kamiko Williams was expected to provide a jolt off the bench on defense, and instead the player she was guarding went around her three consecutive times with little resistance. That parked the junior on the bench for most of the game. Meanwhile, Vicki Baugh was needed inside to counter the size of Vandy, but she was visibly uncomfortable each time she took the floor and went to the locker room once during the game to get treatment. Her left hamstring locked up, shooting pain into her hip and back. "It's hard to play with that," Baugh said. "It's hard to jump. It's hard to move. I tried to play through it. Once it starts there (in the hamstring), it works its way up to my back, hip, and just throws my whole body out of whack. It's unfortunate, but I went through a lot of surgeries and it happens." That left Johnson to handle the duties inside, and once she left the game with foul trouble—she was whistled for two fouls in two seconds in the second half and then fouled out with 5:59 left in the game—the Lady Vols were essentially done.

Balcomb and her players were gracious in the post-game press conference. When Vanderbilt beat Tennessee in the same building in 2009, the celebration continued into the interview room. This was the first win for the Commodores since then, and while they expressed excitement, they also continued to compliment the Lady Vols. In some ways that was understandable, because neither staff would use this game as a defensive tutorial. Tennessee didn't lose the game on offense; 79 points should be enough to beat any team in the SEC. Rather, the Lady Vols lost the game because of lack of defense and rebounds, two staples of any Summitt team.

After the game, a local TV reporter asked Holly Warlick if Summitt had been on the sideline in Memorial Gymnasium for the last time. Warlick seemed momentarily startled—that was the furthest thing from the staff's mind then, and Summitt had publicly said she wanted to continue—but Warlick handled the question well. "I don't think so," she said. "I mean Pat is coaching, she's still coaching, and she's going to continue to coach. So I hope it's not the last time, and I have not heard if it is or isn't. She's still the head coach of this basketball team."

Tennessee had no time to stew over the loss. Kentucky was coming to town for a nationally televised Monday night matchup and had nipped the Lady Vols in Lexington. The Wildcats had started 10–0 in the SEC and had just one conference loss to LSU prior to Tennessee's turn on the schedule on February 13. It was a game that required rubbing one's eyes to adjust to the images—not the Lady Vols running roughshod over a team ranked above them, but the clash of pink and orange. Every shade of pink in the color spectrum was on display from new T-shirts designed for the breast cancer awareness game to older models from past years to the cheerleaders' pompoms to the officials' whistles to the coaches' attire to Tennessee's uniforms to Kentucky's shoes. Mixed in were fans in traditional orange and "We Back Pat" T-shirts and the regular orange outlines of the arena. It was a Crayola moment.

A work of art ended up being painted by the Lady Vols, who, one game after looking inept at times against Vanderbilt, scored the first basket of the game on a long pass from Ariel Massengale to Glory Johnson and never looked back. That the Lady Vols did so with Johnson almost immediately planted on the bench in foul trouble in the first half made the result even more remarkable. Her first foul appeared to be a clean block; her second

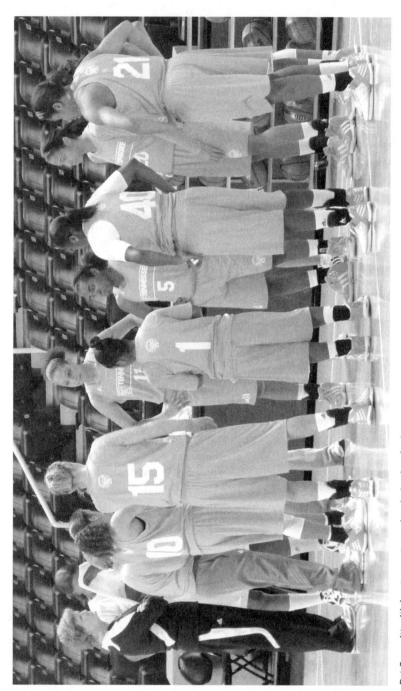

Pat Summitt with her team at practice during her final season.

was a bizarre technical when she tried to save a possession by throwing the ball off a Kentucky player (and missed). Johnson logged just four minutes in the first half, and when she had to leave games, the Lady Vols often unraveled because energy and competitiveness exited with her. But this time with an effective Baugh and additional help from Cierra Burdick and Alicia Manning off the bench, the Lady Vols summoned their inner Glory.

Burdick tallied three boards in five minutes of first-half play. Kamiko Williams grabbed four rebounds in the first half. Added to Baugh's five, that accounted for 12 and allowed Tennessee to wipe out a 15–9 deficit on the glass and finish the half up 20–18, a surge that typically would be unheard of with Johnson reduced to spectator status. "Everyone came in and contributed and that is the kind of effort I expect from a Lady Vol team," Summitt said. "We lost Glory early to fouls and no one hit the panic button. Instead, we had players step up to get the job done. I can't tell you how pleased I was to see that response from our bench." It pleased the crowd, too. They erupted with each basket and clamored for more. They started chants for defense and booed some calls—especially the technical on Johnson—even taking a break for the timeout and restarting their original objection when the game resumed.

The Lady Vols stayed in their 2–3 zone throughout the game, and Kentucky never gave them a reason to come out of it. "I think the last time we played 40 minutes of zone was against Georgia here last year," Warlick said. "As we say, we're a man-to-man team, but we're going to go with what's going to win the game." Despite sticking to the matchup zone, the Lady Vols had 32 points off of Kentucky's 20 miscues. "I am surprised," Warlick said. "But when our zone is active, we create turnovers and it worked for us." Tennessee swamped Kentucky with a 91–54 rout. From the Lady Vol players entering the court via the stands instead of the tunnel to the light shade of pink uniforms, not much resembled the last time Tennessee played at home.

"What a great performance by Tennessee," Kentucky Coach Matthew Mitchell said.

It was a cathartic win for the Lady Vols—and seemingly for their fans, too—after a trying season that reached a low point the week before with a loss to Vanderbilt. "I can tell you our players needed it, our staff needed it, and I'm sure our fans needed this win, too," Summitt said.

21

REGULAR SEASON WINDS DOWN

The much-needed win gave Tennessee a better grip on second place in the SEC with four games to play—two on the road against Mississippi State and Ole Miss and two at home against Arkansas and Florida. But, as always, it's a topsy-turvy league.

The Lady Vols spent most of the regular season's penultimate week in the Magnolia State with a late Thursday evening tipoff in Starkville on February 16, followed by a Sunday afternoon game in Oxford. Tennessee had Taber Spani back on the court, but she was far from healthy, and, unfortunately, had become accustomed to playing that way. Spani endured a freshman season with a painful foot injury that required a summer of rest. She played her sophomore season with an elbow condition that ended up needing surgery. Now, her junior year was severely affected by the bone bruise.

Spani's injuries were unusual. Turf toe is very uncommon among basketball players. She popped out the bursa sac in her elbow while diving for a ball in a preseason drill. The bone bruise occurred during an opposing player's celebration. "It hasn't gotten worse," Spani said. "But it will have to

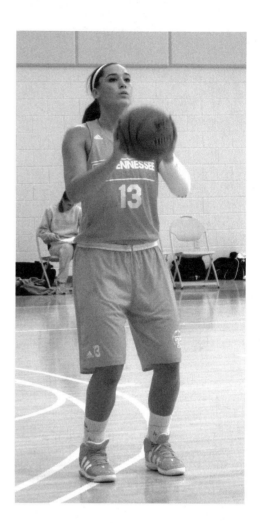

Taber Spani shoots free throws at practice. Pat Summitt's diagnosis devastated the junior guard who chose the Lady Vols because of Summitt.

be after the season to get fully healthy." Spani was Summitt's favorite breed of basketball player—one who never had to be reminded to get in the gym outside of practice to improve her game. But she was forbidden from taking extra shots, because the bone bruise meant she had to rest. Indeed, Spani often used crutches that season off the court, especially when walking to class.

Spani got herself on the court with a Summitt-like sheer force of will. She also tinkered with other aspects of the game to find any advantage. She studied more film with the intent of picking up player tendencies that would help her offensively and defensively. Still, the worst place for an ailing Lady Vol to play was Starkville; matchups with Mississippi State tended to end with players in the training room. The goal of Tennessee in every trip to Starkville had been to get the win and get out of town, and the Lady Vols arrived in 2012 with a 32–0 all-time record against Mississippi State.

The perfect slate for the Lady Vols was not because of lack of defensive effort by the Lady Bulldogs. The games tend to be physical and low scoring, and that was the case again. Vicki Baugh had her mouth bloodied on what was ruled a flagrant foul, though it didn't appear to rise to that level on the replay, and several players on both teams needed a stop in play to restore contacts to their eyes. Any Lady Vol observer expecting a continuation of the fun fest against Kentucky wasn't aware of the history of this series. It was a typical Tennessee-Mississippi State game in that it wasn't pretty to watch. Even steady ball distributor Ariel Massengale had just one credited assist, and baskets were hard to come by on both ends.

Mississippi State played right into Tennessee's hands as the Lady Vols opened in their matchup zone. They didn't play a possession of man defense until three minutes into the second half, and the Lady Bulldogs were content to take—and miss—jump shots. The problem for the Lady Vols was that they were doing the same thing. The two teams combined to shoot 1–20 to open the game. At the 13:40 mark of the first half, Mississippi State led 5–2 on the strength of back-to-back jumpers by Kendra Grant and Diamber Johnson, who hit a trey. "In the beginning we started off really, really well," Grant said. "Everything was flowing and we had the lead at one point. We knew what we had to do in order to beat them. It was a big game and all week we had a saying: 'Shock the world.' That is what we were trying to do." Spani, who didn't appear to be physically comfortable in the game, pulled Tennessee to 5–4 with a middle drive and midrange shot, but the Lady Vol starters, as a whole, continued to sputter.

Enter Baugh, Kamiko Williams and Cierra Burdick.

Baugh got on the glass with five of her six boards coming before halftime, Williams used her ability to create shots to get Mississippi State off balance, and Burdick brought calmness to the floor on offense with her passing and shooting. The trio halted any notion of a shock to the Lady Vols' system, and led by Burdick's 10 points, the Lady Vols' bench outscored Mississippi State's bench 20–0. "I think that's the power of our bench," Holly Warlick said. "Our starters didn't have a particularly good game in the first half." Tennessee played better at high speed and wanted to get its high-octane offense in gear, but the ball squirted loose too frequently with 13 first-half turnovers. "We wanted to pick the pace up and run on them, but we really had a sloppy start," Coach Pat Summitt said.

The Lady Vols got the ball in the hands of Shekinna Stricklen in the second half, and she delivered with 20 second-half points. Tennessee also dominated the glass at 59–37 overall with Stricklen (12 boards) and Glory Johnson (15) leading the way. "I thought Glory and Stricklen did a good job on the boards," Summitt said. "If you can control the boards, you have a great influence on controlling the game." The Magnolia State road swing got off to a great start as Tennessee earned a share of first place in the SEC with the 57–41 victory over Mississippi State and Alabama's upset of Kentucky on the same evening. Tennessee held a workout in Mississippi State's weight room Friday morning, boarded a bus bound for Oxford, and practiced that evening at Ole Miss.

The last time the Lady Vols were in Oxford was February 24, 2011, and the game was halted with a few minutes to play due to inclement weather, and Tennessee leading 66–39. Heavy rain forced its way through the air ducts and deposited itself on the court. After a delay, the conditions were declared unsafe for the players, and the game officially ended. That same location, known as the Tad Pad, was the last road game for the Lady Vols in the 2011–12 season. It was also the last road game in the SEC for five seniors on Tennessee's roster.

One of those was Briana Bass, a point guard from Indianapolis whose arrival in Knoxville coincided with what could be called the Big Experiment at Tennessee: size at all positions and a need to play a lot of zone on defense. The 5'2" Bass saw her playing time diminish as her career unfolded, but she stuck it out and became an integral piece her senior year, bringing energy on defense, pushing the ball in transition, spelling freshman point guard Ariel Massengale, and serving as a leader from the bench. "She is playing the best basketball she's played since she's been at Tennessee, and she is playing with a lot of confidence," Mickie DeMoss said during that road trip. Bass always followed the scouting report on defense, which Warlick praised her for, and she held her own when she was on the court.

That Briana had been able to carve a spot for herself was a credit to her, the staff, and her parents, Tim and Gina Bass. It wasn't an easy process for Briana; she got frustrated and sought counsel from family. "It was tough, but there were four things I always tell her," her father said. "Stay ready, stay hungry, keep working hard, and keep a good attitude. Your team is going to need you." Indeed, Bass was there for her team. She was effective with her minutes and in a teammate's ear with advice or a confidence boost, if needed. "We were always there to pick her up and get her to look at the big picture, but to watch her grow into a leader on this team, even though she doesn't get a lot of minutes, at the end of the day that is what means the most," Tim Bass said.

Briana had expressed interest in becoming a coach and joined the support staff of Indiana women's basketball in 2013. The fans that attended games at Thompson-Boling Arena definitely appreciated her, cheering when she walked to the scorer's table. "I love the support, and I've had the support for four years," she said. When Bass got in the face of an opponent with sticky defense or when she swished a three, the roar in the arena was nearly as loud as if someone in an orange-and-white jersey had just hit a buzzer-beater for the win. "I think when they see Bree's attitude and her smile, I think it's contagious," Tim Bass said. "I just can't believe four years have gone by this fast. I saw my daughter be able to live her dream. Bree's dream was to play at Tennessee and to see that dream fulfilled . . . that is what I tell any kid that is Bree's size or smaller, when you believe in a dream, anything is possible. Dream big." Briana may have been tempted to seek more playing time at another school, but Tim Bass reminded his daughter that the power of sticking with a commitment would pay dividends that may not be readily apparent at first. "I tell people all the time that is how a seed grows," he said. "It grows when you keep it in place."

The Lady Vols completed the state sweep of Mississippi and returned home still competing for first place in the SEC with a 66–56 win over Ole Miss. The victory was No. 20 on the season, a milestone Tennessee reached for 36 consecutive years under Pat Summitt. While neither game in the Magnolia State was particularly pretty, the coaches would take the victories. Nikki Byrd, one of three Rebel seniors honored before the game, wore a "We Back Pat" T-shirt at the center court ceremony, as did seniors Whitney Hamath and LaTosha Laws.

By late February, teams are just trying to survive conference play and get into postseason intact. The Lady Vols spent five days in Mississippi and were ready to return to Knoxville, sleep in their own beds, catch up with school, and get in the gym on their own time.

But Mississippi wasn't quite ready for Summitt to leave. Tennessee and Ole Miss fans gathered near the team bus, and Summitt kept signing autographs even after the bus was loaded and ready to depart. As was often the case, Meshia Thomas was nearby. Thomas was getting signals from athletics administrators to get Summitt on the bus, but Summitt said no and kept signing. "I can't override no," said Thomas, who said the signals turned into looks of demand from the administrators. Thomas had to take the pen from Summitt in that case to get the head coach to the bus so the team could get to the airport and finally get back to Tennessee after nearly a week in hotel rooms. "My job was to try to keep people at bay, but it's very difficult to do that when she wanted to give autographs. I would get looks from other people in athletics like, 'Why are you letting her do this?' She didn't want to say no."

Thomas was used to the crowds. It happened everywhere Summitt went, especially during that final season. Most of the time Summitt followed Thomas' cues about when to leave. Other times, she kept the Sharpie and signed away. "Sometimes I was saying no and she would go, 'Yes.' And behind that she would call me boss lady," Thomas said. "I said, 'OK, you're trying to be funny. Because you're calling me boss lady but then you're doing the opposite of what I am telling you to do.' We really had a great relationship."

The Lady Vols were in great shape in the SEC with two games to play and certainly didn't want to stumble at home. First up was Arkansas, which had won nine of its past 10 games after a horrid start in the SEC. "I am very impressed with what they've done," Dean Lockwood said two days before the February 23 game. "They have my full respect. That was a fork in the road for them. They could have tanked. They really regrouped. I respect this team a great deal."

Tennessee would close the regular season with Senior Day on February 26 against Florida. The Gators had just defeated Georgia to even their SEC record and were making a late season case for an NCAA Tournament berth. The SEC was better in 2011–12 and was already likely to get at least six teams—maybe eight—in the NCAA tourney, with Arkansas and Florida making their statements. "They are one of the scrappiest teams in the league right now," Lockwood said of Florida. "They don't die. You've got to shoot them five times in the head, cut their head off, set them on fire and then maybe, maybe, maybe they're dead. They just don't die. I love that about them."

Tennessee had its share of challenges in the SEC and had already been tagged with three losses against Kentucky, South Carolina, and Vanderbilt. Even the wins felt like alley fights most of the time. "That is how I feel," Lockwood said. "I feel like every game is a brawl. I think the talent level is probably as evenly distributed as it's been in some time. I think there are some programs that have been building and now they've turned a corner. This league has gotten to the point where the top five, six, you might as well flip a coin on a given night."

It was a special week for Baugh. Her grandparents, Calvin and Barbara Baugh, arrived in town from Sacramento and would see their granddaughter play in Knoxville for the first time in her career. Barbara Baugh, who was at practice wearing a No. 21 pin, was last in Tennessee when her granddaughter had her second ACL surgery. She saw a Lady Vols game during that 2009 trip, but this time she finally got to see Baugh play on "The Summitt" floor. Baugh's grandparents remained in town for the Senior Day game, too. "This is their first game where I will be playing in a game," Baugh said. "I am just excited that they are here. I am showing them Knoxville. They love it." Baugh turned a corner in February mentally and physically, playing well in back-to-back games on the road and seeming more comfortable on the court.

"We have yet to play our best basketball," Lockwood said. "We can be a lot better. We can reach deeper." It started with the team's output of energy. "I call it the sense of urgency that everything is important," Lockwood said. "It's kind of like a firehouse when the bell rings. They're not wild but there's a sense of purpose. Those guys know that in seven seconds I've got to be down a pole, geared up and on a truck when somebody's life is on the line. That is kind of what we're looking for. We want a sense of urgency that every possession is important. Every little thing that happens we attach value to it."

Tennessee had energy to spare when it hosted Kentucky, and the result was the 91–54 romp. The first time the Lady Vols played Arkansas they followed the scouting report to a T and posted a 69–38 win in Fayetteville, but Arkansas arrived in Knoxville a vastly improved team since that January 8 game. The Razorbacks were seeking their first-ever program win in Knoxville. "We have a lot of confidence but we know that Knoxville is a tough place to play and win, but we are eager to go in and redeem ourselves and play well," Arkansas Coach Tom Collen said. Lockwood expected a stiff test from the Razorbacks, who were building a resume for inclusion in the NCAA Tournament. They entered the last week of the regular season in a four-team tie for third place in the SEC with Georgia, LSU, and South Carolina.

Noting the erratic starts from game to game, the Tennessee coaches tried different approaches, but nothing had clicked yet. "We've hammered; we've backed off a little bit," Lockwood said. "We're searching for the magical note. We're playing all the keys, hitting them lightly, hitting them firmly and we haven't hit that magical note." Tennessee didn't want to hit a sour note against Arkansas. The Lady Vols ended up having to expend a lot of energy to get ahead in the game. They led 7–5 on a baseline jumper from Meighan

Simmons at the 17:02 mark of the first half and then didn't lead again until Taber Spani connected on two free throws for a 46–44 score with 11:30 to play, which energized the crowd of 13,337.

With 1:05 remaining, Tennessee clung to a four-point lead, 62–58, after Kamiko Williams grabbed an offensive board and hit the stick-back in one motion and Shekinna Stricklen connected on a turn-around. But Arkansas came back with two layups from C'eira Ricketts and Sarah Watkins to force an extra five minutes. Ricketts scored a layup in overtime, and Arkansas built a six-point lead, 70–64, with 1:55 left after Calli Berna connected on her only trey of the game. Stricklen answered with a three to trim the lead to 70–67, and then—after Arkansas' fifth shot clock violation of the game—she scored on a putback to pull Tennessee within one point, 70–69, with 45 seconds left.

After a Razorback turnover out of bounds, Stricklen brought the ball down court and was fouled by Keira Peak. But Stricklen missed both—she had missed two from the stripe earlier in the extra period—and Lyndsay Harris connected on two free throws for a 72–69 lead with 6.2 seconds left. Ariel Massengale was fouled with three seconds left before Tennessee could launch a three, and she made the first free throw to trim the lead to 72–70. She intended to miss the second, but it swished through the net. "I was trying to," Massengale said. "Coach told me right when the ref gave it to me to shoot it quick and just try to hit it off the rim and get the rebound. Unfortunately, it went in. I was trying to shoot it off to the right so Glory could hopefully get the rebound and put it back in."

Simmons nearly got a steal, but Dominique Robinson went to the line for Arkansas with 2.6 seconds left. She missed both, but Stricklen's last-second shot hit the front iron and the Lady Vols fell 72–71. Stricklen crumpled to the court and was still visibly upset in the post-game press conference. "I have to sink the free throws," Stricklen said in a barely audible voice. "I honestly wanted the ball at the end. I clearly missed four free throws in a row. One could've given us the lead to the game. One could've tied up the game. We had a bad first half, but we came back in the second half. We fought."

The Lady Vols lost their third game at home—a program record in one season. "Give Arkansas all the credit," Summitt said. "There is a reason why they have been the hottest team in our conference over the last month. Their entire team played well, but we basically let three Arkansas players beat us—Lyndsay Harris, Sarah Watkins, and C'eira Ricketts." Massengale sat at the table with two seniors, who now had just one home game left in their careers. Both of the seniors looked emotionally spent. Massengale, who had six assists and was one away from tying Loree Moore's rookie record of 133, remained composed. "We've told Strick that we don't lose games off the last play," Massengale said. "It hurts that she missed those free throws, but I think as a team we lost that game for ourselves right from the get-go. We just didn't come out with the right mindset that I think we should have."

That had been a season-long issue for Tennessee, and the coaches went 11 deep in the first half with Williams, Baugh, and Cierra Burdick scoring four points each to keep Tennessee within five at halftime, when the Razorbacks led 31–26. Tennessee shot 45 percent in the first half, but Arkansas scorched the nets at 57.9 percent, including 5–10 from long range. "When you shoot 45 percent the first half, you think you're doing well," Warlick said. "But they were shooting 58 percent. So at one point you've got to say the defense has to step up and make stops, and we didn't make stops the first half. So, we dug ourselves a hole."

Arkansas worked deep into the shot clock—the Razorbacks had four shot clock violations in the first half—and kept the ball in the hands of Ricketts, Watkins, and Harris for the most part. "I wanted to do that in Fayetteville but when we did that in Fayetteville and then we missed shots, we weren't very successful," Collen said. "In some ways I was a little bit hesitant to come back and try to play that way, but I think the tradeoff was that we controlled the pace of the game that way. We had the ball in our best players' hands that way. It hasn't always worked but tonight it worked."

Neither Warlick nor the Lady Vol players was at a loss for words after the game. They outlined what went wrong, what they should have done differently, and how they can't start games slowly and always expect to recover. But it didn't necessarily mean that the lesson would stick. "It is frustrating because I know their ability and what they can do," Warlick said. "And they battled. We just continued to dig ourselves a hole and we've got to climb out of it. So if we can ever put together a 40-minute game—I love this team. When they're all clicking, it's a great group. We just have lapses and we've got to get to a point where we close those lapses and shorten those lapses."

It was the fourth loss in the league this season with two preseason All-SEC First Team members in Stricklen and Glory Johnson. Johnson was saddled with two fouls in the first half and didn't score or get a board in eight minutes. Stricklen logged 10 minutes before halftime and also didn't score or get a rebound. They are the ones who set the tone. "It was awful," Johnson said by way of describing the first half. "I went out with two fouls. We weren't hitting shots that we should have hit. We had no energy at all. We had to go to our bench, and then all of the sudden they're out-rebounding us. We were letting them penetrate in the paint, and they shouldn't be in the paint. We weren't playing our game, and you see that with us a lot. Sometimes we play great first half and awful second half. We always try to pick it up late in the game, but we're just not a team that can do that. It just doesn't work out that way for us."

There was nothing ambiguous in that answer, which Johnson expanded on without prompting. She immediately identified what happened and what should not have occurred, and it had all been said before. What the team hadn't been able to do was cycle out of its loop of inconsistency. There were some legitimate reasons for their struggles. They hadn't been healthy for four years. Baugh played an effective eight minutes in the first half but seemed visibly uncomfortable on the bench before the second half started. It would be an ideal time to set a regular starting lineup and rotation, but the coaches don't always know until game day—and in Baugh's case, in game—who would be available. Meighan Simmons logged just 15 minutes and a player who essentially had no restrictions placed on her as a freshman found herself at the opposite extreme as a sophomore, with quick hooks and long stretches on the bench.

Lockwood had specifically mentioned energy and the fact it had to be present from the get-go for this team to succeed. The players said it was essential to their success, yet Stricklen and Johnson became spectators in the first half because they combined for zero points and zero boards in 18 combined minutes of play. "Obviously, I wish I could explain why we came out flat, but I have no idea why we came out the way we did," Summitt said. "The coaching staff wishes we had an answer."

Another thing Summitt had been seeking an answer for was why she had to constantly remind players to get extra shots on their own. She couldn't force them, and it had been an ongoing struggle to get the team, as a whole, to do so for the past four years. Freshman Cierra Burdick noted on a post-game radio show that the players needed to find the ball racks. When a freshman points that out to a team with seven juniors and seniors, it indicates a major flaw in a team's makeup. Still, the Lady Vols had time. And they definitely had the talent. Johnson had put together a league MVP quality season.

Stricklen shook off a bad first half and tallied 17 points. The usually dependable free throw shooter missed four from the stripe in overtime.

If Stricklen connected on those, the storyline became one of resilience and overcoming a scorching hot team, not one of outlining how the Lady Vols succumbed again at home. Such is the thin line of sports narratives.

Warlick made it clear how much the staff liked this team. In three days, the coaches and fans would say goodbye to a senior class that had endured more than any group in the history of the program from nearly losing a teammate to a brain aneurysm to finding out before the season started that Summitt had early onset dementia. From that point of view, they had persevered. On the flip side, Summitt still had to remind players to get in the gym on their own. That lesson—especially given the shooting percentages at times that season—should have already stuck, and the fact it had not was baffling.

But there was this to consider: the exhaustion, both physical and emotional, of players undergoing a season while watching a titan of the game have to take a vastly different role within the program she built from scratch. "It was really tough, because Holly was trying to protect Pat and look out for the best interests of Pat, and Mickie was trying to protect Pat and look out for the best interests of Pat," Johnson said. "And Pat was looking to her assistant coaches to make the decisions. We tried to stick together. It was really, really tough for everybody."

The fact that the players cared was not in dispute, nor should it ever be. Stricklen collapsed to the floor after the Arkansas game ended and dissolved into tears. Williams had to help her up, and Baugh put an arm around her as they headed to the locker room. "It's not her fault," Johnson said. "Clearly we played an awful first half. There were so many mistakes made in the first half like missing free throws. I missed two free throws. The blame is not on her. It's a team game."

And, once again, as a team they still had time. The clock on the 2011–12 season continued to tick.

22

SENIOR DAY

S enior Day usually means a shift in the starting lineup. Pat Summitt
always started seniors for their last home game. Seniors are often already starters, but if not, the reserves become starters on their day to be
recognized.

Summitt had five seniors to honor on February 26, 2012, when they
would play their final game on "The Summitt" court on a Sunday afternoon.
Losing a quintet at one time would be a blow to the roster the next season.
"It's pretty hard to see them all leave because they've done a great job here,"
Summitt said during media interviews that week. "They've all been invested.
I think come Senior Day, we're all going to look around and say, 'What hap-
pened?'" Sunday's matchup with Florida was an important one. The Gators
needed to boost their NCAA resume, same as Arkansas, and had five seniors
of their own. The Gators' largest margin of defeat was just 14 points against
Rutgers. The other nine losses had all been by six points or less.

The uncertainty of Summitt's health going forward meant it was possible
that Sunday was Summitt's final home game as head coach, and the players

were well aware of the speculation. The Lady Vols had to somehow set aside the emotion of Senior Day and get ready for tipoff. It became a defining moment of the season, and more than 17,000 tickets were sold in advance for the final home game. Some years Tennessee is a host site for the early rounds of the NCAA Tournament, but that wasn't the case in 2012, so it really would be the final game of the 2011–12 season. "Give them something to remember," Glory Johnson said. "They won't get to see us again on that home floor."

Five seniors provided a ready-made lineup to honor the veterans. Johnson and Shekinna Stricklen were regular starters, Alicia Manning had 10 nods that season, and Vicki Baugh had 11. It was Briana Bass' second start of the season, but she had held her own during minutes off the bench. Bass had logged 11 minutes against Arkansas and graded out very high on the game film. "She did exactly what she was asked to do and the way she was asked to do it," Dean Lockwood said. "She was getting to (C'eria Ricketts). I get fired up by that stuff. You annoy. You disrupt. You bother."

The coaches had sought a starting five all season that could consistently get the team off to a high-energy start, and they thought they had finally turned the corner in the rout over Kentucky. But with the same opening players, both road games in Mississippi started slowly, the coaches were forced to go to the bench early, and then the sputtering continued at home against Arkansas. "We're looking for a mode of play," Lockwood said. "This is what you're going to get when you hit the court. It's competing and a focus and an awareness level. We have been searching for a unit." That meant three regular starters in freshman Ariel Massengale, sophomore Meighan Simmons, and junior Taber Spani would come off the bench on Senior Day. The five seniors would likely shed some tears and then focus the way Lockwood mentioned.

The way Stricklen saw it, if Manning and Bass didn't start crying, she would hold back the tears, too. The way all of them saw it, if their family members got emotional, they would likely join them in needing some tissues before tipoff. "It will be a pretty emotional day because we all worked our whole lives to play here," Manning said. It was also a longer ceremony than in recent years. Three years previously in 2009, only one senior departed; in 2010 there were none; and in 2011 there were two. The original class arrived as a crew of six, but two members departed—Amber Gray transferred to Xavier in her home state of Ohio to be close to her physicians, and Alyssia Brewer transferred to UCLA before the 2011–12 season began.

The class added a member in Baugh, the fifth-year redshirt who underwent two ACL surgeries on her left knee and earned a national title ring as a true freshman. "I am kind of like the mom to them, but at the same time those are my girls because we're all seniors together," Baugh said. "But I call myself the super senior just because I've got that extra little bit of knowledge. I am going to be losing my sisters, but the beauty of Tennessee is that we will remain family off the court." It was a class that has endured to say the least. Off the court, they survived the near-death of Gray, staff member Daedra Charles-Furlow's battle with breast cancer, the exit of teammates to transfer and major injury, and the thunderbolt before the season began that Summitt had early onset dementia.

On the court, they were still seeking their first Final Four, their NCAA resume included the program's first-ever first round loss, and they lost more games at home this season than any Lady Vol team ever had. "Our class has been through a lot with the four years that we have been here and then what happened this summer with Pat," Stricklen said. "It brought everyone close, the team and coaches." The Tennessee coaches wanted the seniors to savor that Sunday's ceremony. "I hope they have a moment of thankfulness and gratitude," Lockwood said. "I hope they can enjoy the fact of playing at a place this special and this unique."

The seniors were asked before that game how they would sort out their emotions. "I don't know if I might cry or not," Baugh said. "I don't know what my emotions will be. I just know that this program has truly been a huge piece of my heart." Stricklen chose not to think about it too much. "It still hasn't hit me yet," Stricklen said. "It probably won't hit me until that Sunday. Tears? Only if I see the rest of them crying. I am going to try not to look at Bree or A-Town (Alicia Manning) because I know those two will."

"I'm determined not to cry," Bass said. "After the game I am probably going to have some boohoo moments. As long as I don't look at anybody crying I will be fine. I appreciate this experience. We don't talk about it being over. We don't want to look at it as being over."

The pre-game ceremony took about 15 minutes as the Lady Vols said goodbye to three managers, two student trainers, and five basketball players, and the crowd of 18,563 seemed to savor every second of it. Summitt, as always, handed flowers to all of them and posed for individual and group photos. When it was time for the starting lineups, Summitt, as always, presented the five Florida seniors with flowers, too.

Gator guard Jordan Jones, who is from Suwanee, Georgia, gave Summitt a big hug while taking her flowers and spoke to the head coach before returning to the bench. "Every kid grows up, especially in the South, watching Pat Summitt," Jones said. "She is the reason why I am playing basketball.

She really got this game started for us, and I can't say enough about the amount of respect that I have for her. I told her that since they announced the news I have been praying for her and the team every night and that she is an inspiration to everyone. That is exactly what I said, and I mean every word of it."

It was that kind of pre-game ceremony, and then a basketball contest had to be played. Jones got Florida on the scoreboard first with a deep three ball, and then Tennessee went on a 15–0 run to open the game. "We knew that they were going to come out intense, fiery," Jones said. "That's on us that we didn't respond, answer the way we have all season long. Honestly, we start slow a lot and normally we're able to bounce back; against a great team like Tennessee and on their home court, it is not possible to do." Tennessee had had its issues with slow starts that season, but the five seniors changed the script for their final game at Thompson-Boling Arena. "All five of our seniors came ready to play and got off to a good start," Summitt said. "That was really important for this team."

Manning set the tone on both ends. She nailed a three, got on the boards, shared the ball, and disrupted Florida on defense. "She was relaxed and she played her game," Holly Warlick said. "She wasn't forcing things, she wasn't trying to make things happen—the game came to her. And when she lets that come to her, she's a heck of a player." Manning logged 14 minutes in the first half and combined with Johnson to score 15 of the Lady Vols' first 17 points. When the first substitute entered—Cierra Burdick nine minutes into the first half—Tennessee had built a 17–8 lead and Florida had used two timeouts.

The coaches liked the high energy to open the game from Bass getting a steal and flipping the ball back in-bounds to Manning, who found Stricklen for a layup, to Stricklen saving a loose ball at Tennessee's end and sending it between a Florida player's legs to Bass, who found Johnson. The crowd responded to hustle plays with the same enthusiasm they gave for made baskets. "We have the best fans in America," Holly Warlick said. "And regardless of what situation we're dealing with, our fans came out to support our team and our coaching staff. We have five seniors and I didn't expect anything less. This year, they seem to be really into the game more, and I love it. I love when they get on the officials; I love when they get into it. It's just a great thing to see our fans have a lot of respect for our seniors."

That was an accurate observation.

When games got tight that season, the fans got more engaged and even louder. Perhaps they sensed that this team needed even more support. On that Sunday they were thunderous in their applause for each senior. "The Lady Vol fans have always had our back whether we're winning or losing," Johnson said. "They're always staying positive with us; you've got to love it. That's what we came here for. That's what we expect from our fans." Fans sat in the very back rows of the upper reaches of the arena and packed the lower bowl. With the uncertainty of Summitt's health going forward, fans were also there to see the final home game of the season and what they thought could be Summitt's last game in the arena as head coach.

"I don't think so," Johnson said afterwards. "We don't know anything about that. If she was going to do that, she would've let us know. She was just really happy to be there, and we were happy to have her there. Until she says when, we're going to keep on being happy." Amid that backdrop, the Lady Vols had to focus on the game. That had been difficult for them at times, but that afternoon, led by the seniors, they seemed to embrace the challenge. The coaches used nine players in the first half—double digits for all five seniors with the other minutes spread among Massengale, Simmons, Burdick, and Spani. The result was a 10-point lead (35–25) at halftime that ended with Massengale zipping the ball down court and finding Johnson at the rim.

The seniors opened the second half, too, and Baugh found Manning, who curled the ball to Johnson for a layup 16 seconds into the half for a 37–25 lead. Stricklen got on track from long range during the second half and hit three treys. Manning had a hand in Stricklen's first three-pointer when she got the miss and got the ball right back to Stricklen, who buried the three on the second try for a 43–30 lead. After Manning got a highlight block on the other end, she got the ball to Stricklen in the corner for a 46–32 lead. "A couple of her threes were really timely," Summitt said. They were indeed, because Florida stayed in striking distance until the final two minutes when Massengale hit a pair of free throws with 2:20 left to put the lead in double digits for good, 68–57. Simmons and Massengale also connected from the field to keep Florida at bay. Tennessee closed its scoring with a nearly length-of-the-court, in-bounds pass to Johnson from Manning, a Massengale drive that found Manning, and a Stricklen free throw. Then, three of the seniors, Johnson and Manning first and then Stricklen, left to standing ovations in the final minute. Massengale drove and dished to Isabelle Harrison for the final 75–59 score. The seniors walked off their home court for the last time as victors.

All 10 available Lady Vols logged minutes in the game. Junior guard Kamiko Williams was held out for medical reasons, but was going to be available for postseason. Manning had an impressive stat line for her Senior Day—11 points, eight boards, six assists, three steals, and a block. "I was just excited, and our fans have just been with us through everything," Manning said. "I personally felt like I owed it to them. I owed it to my family. They're the reason I'm here." Perhaps the most impressive thing about Johnson's stat line was zero fouls in 37 minutes, despite a physical game in the post. "That was the first thing I screamed when I went into the locker room was that I had zero fouls, and I was so happy," Johnson said. "Games like that are where you kind of stay composed and let the refs handle it."

Tennessee played in Summitt's image to close the regular season. Her impact on the game extended to the Gators, who wore "We Back Pat" T-shirts during warm-ups. Jones had hers on for the post-game press conference, too.

"We're trying to show as much support as we can for the greatest coach in women's basketball history," Jones said.

Tennessee also finally found a starting lineup in its last regular season game. The five seniors took the floor and started the game just as the coaches had hoped they would: with high energy on both ends. "Right now they're our starting five unless it proves something different in practice the next couple of days," Warlick said. "They got us off to a great start and they had a lot of pride in wearing the Tennessee orange." The entire program—seniors, teammates, coaches, and support staff—needed the win. It helped to erase the bitterness of the loss to Arkansas, which allowed Kentucky to win the SEC outright rather than share it with Tennessee as co-champs. The Lady Vols earned the No. 2 seed for the upcoming SEC tourney. "All I wanted to do was get a win and go into the SEC Tournament on a positive note," Warlick said. "We created our own fate, and we've got to live with it."

Warlick was visibly relieved at the post-game press conference. She entered after the previous game looking beleaguered, but this time, she was smiling and didn't look as if she had played for 40 minutes. "I obviously loved it," Warlick said. "I was really, really excited for the seniors. And as much as they've taken a lot of heat from a lot of situations, I'm extremely proud of them." When Warlick was asked about Massengale setting the freshman assist record—Loree Moore had 133; Massengale now has 137—the associate head coach (and former Lady Vol point guard) cracked up the room with her response. "Where am I on that ranking?" Warlick asked. "I'd have pulled her right on out."

Florida Coach Amanda Butler was asked if SEC post players would welcome the end of Johnson's eligibility. Johnson frustrated every Gator who tried to guard her and finished with 21 points and 10 boards. "Post players, coaches, and guards," Butler said of the list that was glad to see Johnson graduate. "She is a great representative of our league, and I think it is one of the reasons you choose this league as a competitor because you want to either play with or against the Glory Johnsons. She is a fantastic representative of the SEC and certainly of the University of Tennessee, a great competitor, and she is just hard to handle. It's really hard to guard her one-on-one. She has made the most of her career here. I think there will be some graduation gifts sent to her for sure."

Johnson is of slender build, definitely better suited to power forward, but played the bulk of her Lady Vol career at center because of injuries to other post players. She answered the bell for every single game in her career and had now played in 135 games with 112 starts. "As long as I keep playing big, I don't care what size I am, how much I weigh, I'm going to keep playing as big as I can play," Johnson said. That was advice the entire senior class had to absorb. It was a class that had been through hell and back with no bigger blow than the sucker punch that landed in late summer with the news about Summitt.

On the court this season, they absorbed more punches with eight losses, including four in the SEC. But on Senior Day all five lined up for the opening tip and then did exactly what the coaches asked on both ends of the court. "It comes down to us just setting our minds to it really," said Manning, who unleashed her inner senior. "It just can't be four people on the floor. It can't be three people on the floor. It's got to be all five, and the bench has got to be ready whenever their number is called, so it's got to be a collective effort, and it's got to be a sense of urgency all the time." It was a class that had been much maligned for what it had done—first round loss in the NCAA tourney in 2009—and for what it had not done—reached a Final Four.

Let the seniors write the ending. Their team, their legacy.

23

PAT SUMMITT'S BODYGUARD

Meshia Thomas was an officer with the UT Police Department, but because she was seen so often next to Summitt, she became indelibly linked to the head coach. Head coaches are usually escorted during games at home and on the road, and when Thomas was selected to provide security for Summitt, it wasn't her first close encounter with the icon. Thomas had played basketball in high school in Jesup, Georgia, and walked on at Tennessee State University in Nashville. Thomas had some scholarship offers, but she was attracted to TSU because she ran track as well—and it was the alma mater of her idol, Wilma Rudolph, who she got to meet at the school.

She would later leave Nashville for Knoxville, where she had some friends from high school who were now at Knoxville College. They encouraged Thomas, a post player, to join the team, which had just five players at the time. "I was the sixth one," said Thomas, who played for two semesters during the 1994–95 season. A highlight that year was a game against Maryville College to be played at Thompson-Boling Arena. Maryville

College, located just 17 miles from Tennessee's campus, was coached by former Lady Vol Kelli Casteel Cook. "This is my first time in Thompson-Boling Arena, ever," Thomas said. "We walk in with our little bags. Six players. I had never seen anything like this in my life. I was blown away at the crowd and the excitement."

The Lady Vols played the first game of a double-header; Maryville College and Knoxville College played the second game. "My coach kept saying, 'You're going to play in front of Coach Summitt.' I said, 'She is not going to watch our game,'" Thomas said. When the Knoxville College players went to warm up for their game, the crowd had dwindled but Summitt and Jenny Moshak remained in the arena, despite the lopsided score, as Maryville College cruised to a win. "I got hurt during that game," Thomas said. "I took a really bad fall. Went up for a rebound, feet went up one way, and feet came down last." Moshak checked on Thomas. And then Summitt went to the bench to chat with her.

"Coach came over and talked to me. She said, 'Hey, what's your name?' I was about to pass out at that point. She said, 'You're jumping out of the gym. How much eligibility do you have?' I said, 'Unfortunately, Coach, this is it for me. I started back in this a little late.'" Thomas was 23 then, and "I wasn't trying to set any records for being the oldest collegiate player playing the sport." Thomas was ready to start her work career after basketball ended. She had experience in sales and management and was working in customer service for a cable company when she saw an opening for a UT police dispatcher, applied, and got the entry-level job.

"I was at the school where you had the winningest basketball team in the country," Thomas said. "When I thought about a basketball team growing up, it was the Lady Vols. It was Pat Summitt. I thought, 'What a great opportunity to be at the same school. Maybe I will run into her.'" Thomas performed well in the dispatcher position, and police officers told her that she had the demeanor to be on patrol. Thomas graduated from the police academy and became a police officer. Her assignments included working at some Lady Vol games at the arena, where she saw Summitt. "I stood back in awe and just watched at a distance."

Summitt had noticed Thomas at those games, and she wanted her assigned to Lady Vol security. The 2007 team had won a national title. Candace Parker and crew were superstars, and the head coach saw a need for enhanced protection of her players, especially in postseason with extended hotel stays. Thomas had a commanding presence about her—no-nonsense and authoritative on-duty but with a warm smile when warranted. Thomas was also African American, as were the majority of the Tennessee players. That wasn't lost on Summitt. She wanted positive role models for her players, and an accomplished black woman was a perfect fit for the team.

Thomas came aboard in 2008, which culminated with a national title in Tampa. The post-game trophy presentation was in the NCAA hotel, a downtown Hyatt, which was also where the Lady Vols stayed for the Final Four. Summitt was very superstitious. "We were walking through the hotel back to her room and she looked at me and said, 'Well, we won, so I'll just have to keep taking you with me,'" Thomas said. Summitt was quite serious. UT police officers shifted into different departmental positions, but whenever it was suggested that Thomas make a move, the head coach nixed it. "They like consistency," Thomas said of the Lady Vols program. "Pat said, 'We're going to keep you.'"

Thomas moved through the ranks into supervisory positions. "I actually at one point tried to back out because I thought I needed to put more emphasis on that. But it wasn't happening, according to Coach Summitt. She made up her mind, and I followed suit. I got a chance to get a lot closer to her." Thomas' face became familiar to fans at games and on television, because she was always close by while also trying to stay out of the spotlight.

On February 5, 2009, Summitt parked under Pratt Pavilion as usual and headed into the arena for a game against Georgia. Media greeted her. It wasn't a standard SEC game during the regular season; Summitt had 999 career wins, and a victory that evening would be No. 1,000. "Everybody was prepared for that," Thomas said. "You've got cameras everywhere. When her car pulls to her spot, she gets out, they put cameras on her catching her every moment."

Thomas hovered but stood out of the range of the camera frames, which had tightened on Summitt. The head coach was always accessible to the media, and she smiled at all the attention. "I felt like, 'This is your big day.' I backed off. Give her space. She's walking in like the queen that she is of women's basketball," Thomas said. "I've got my cell phone, and I am sending messages through work. I didn't realize that she stopped still in her tracks, so I almost bumped into her. I stop and she is right there. She is looking at me with these eyes and she says, 'What are you doing?' I said, 'Uh . . . Coach . . . nothing.' She said, 'Get up here by me. This is where you are supposed to be.' I said, 'Coach, this is your big day. I will follow you. I will pay attention. I will put my phone away.' She laughed and said, 'No, this is our day.' That will forever be etched into my brain. She always made me feel like I was part of the Lady Vol family."

After getting the job as Summitt's bodyguard, as she came to be called, one of Thomas' first road trips with Tennessee was to Oklahoma for the NCAA regional in Oklahoma City. She was in the lobby of the hotel waiting for the players as they came down to get ready for a bus ride to practice. "I was trying to build a relationship with the players," she said. Jenny Moshak arrived and challenged Thomas to an arm wrestling contest—the uber-fit athletic trainer vs. the police officer. Both women are also very competitive. "The team is going for Jenny. Nobody is going for me. Nobody. We are locked up it seemed like forever. And I can see her turning colors. I think, 'If I can just stay locked up, she'll give'. We stayed locked up, and I won. That was the pivotal point. The kids were like, 'Oh, my God, you're strong?' I was like, 'I can hold my own.' At that point they were like, 'Oh, you're a bodyguard. We trust you. You can take care of us.'"

Summitt trusted Thomas to take care of her players. When Angie Bjorklund came home to a ransacked apartment—though nothing was taken—she called her head coach, who told her to immediately call 911.

Summitt then called Thomas, who was at home off-duty at the time, and asked her to get to the complex. Thomas didn't hesitate to respond. "She said, 'Angie thinks someone is in her apartment or has been in her apartment.'" While driving to the apartment, Thomas saw a vehicle, which contained Lady Vol players, going past her in the opposite direction. They called Thomas, doubled back, and met her at the entrance.

"Angie hasn't seen me at this point. They said, 'We just want to let you know it was a prank. She should have known it! Our stuff was there!' I am like, 'Are you serious?' I got back in my car, rolled the window up, and I started to call Coach. And they are standing outside of my window with these faces like, 'Are you calling her?' I rolled my window down. I said, 'She already knows. She called me!' So, I called Coach and put her mind at ease. It was indeed a joke, and no one is injured. Of course, Coach was not happy. She said, 'What do you want to do?' I said, 'I'm going to make them clean it up.' She said, 'OK, call me before you leave.' And they are still trembling basically. I said, 'Let's go up here. You guys are coming with me.'"

A Knoxville Police Department officer was already on the scene following the 911 call, and Thomas identified herself to him. She explained the "break-in" was a prank and identified the "culprits," who were there to clean up the apartment. Thomas was annoyed because she knew police resources had been used to answer the call, but the officer smiled and decided that would resolve the case. The team was leaving for the SEC tourney in Nashville shortly thereafter, so the players were understandably uptight about seeing Summitt. "She made some comments about it on the bus." Thomas said. "They were nervous. That look scares me. I would not have been a part of that prank. I would have been like, 'Sorry, guys, I am out.' It could have been a worse prank, but having the police there wasn't a good thing because he could have been responding to something more important. But he was fine with it so it turned out OK."

Thomas also stepped in when Tyler Summitt neglected to pay some parking tickets. His mother learned about it from her son shortly before a game. The fact it was Tyler on the phone was one of the few reasons the head coach would take a call that close to tipoff. "She got a phone call right before she is getting ready to walk out on the court," Thomas said. "She is talking to Tyler on the phone. I realized it was him because of what she was saying, the stern look, and she was giving me the look. So I knew it was bad. She kept saying, 'You don't do things like that. You are held to a higher standard.' She gives me the phone and says, 'Here, Meshia, talk to Tyler.'"

A very subdued Tyler was on the other end of the phone. "I said, 'Bring your checkbook,'" said Thomas, who also advised Tyler to go to parking services and select a parking plan. "It wasn't, 'Oh, let me take care of that for you.' That is not Coach Summitt's way. Coach Summitt is about responsibility. I wasn't going to give him an out." Tyler laughs about it now. "Oh, my gosh, that was absolutely funny. Mom didn't miss anything. I always wondered how she knew things but I came to realize someone would always update her. Her players were always like, 'How does she know about everything? She knows about things before I even do them?' I went right away—trust me."

Thomas didn't just provide security for Summitt; her role was also one as a UTPD liaison for the players. She created parameters for standards of behavior with responsibility topping the list. She told them how to handle tickets—as Tyler knows, that means pay them—and retrieve towed vehicles. At one meeting, some players asked about parking tickets issued by the Knoxville Police Department, which, unlike the UTPD, can't withhold transcripts and such until they are paid. They quizzed Thomas about various scenarios, including tickets issued to the car's actual owner, such as their parents. "They kept coming with the 'what ifs.' Coach popped up and said, 'I am tired of this. This is not a 'what if.' If you are playing for this program, you are going to be responsible for what you do. Period.' It was that look of we're done with this."

At Summitt's behest, Thomas discussed safety programs, community awareness, and places to avoid because their presence there would reflect poorly on the team, something that became especially important in the age of smartphones and social media. "Sometimes I was the bad guy, but I think most of the time I was able to get the point across where they trusted I was being honest," Thomas said. "I felt more like a mom than a police officer. She would tell them, 'You had better listen to what Meshia has to say.'"

Summitt always made sure that Thomas was accepted and treated with respect, and that extended to big donor events at her home. "It was like she was zoned on me and she wanted to make sure that I was OK," Thomas said. "She came up to me, 'Are you good? Remember, you don't have to be the police. Just mingle. These are friends.' I appreciated that. It was all about, 'This can help you. These people might be able to help you.'" This exposure gave Thomas a foothold in the community, and she served on boards for the Sexual Assault Crisis Center and the Sertoma Center. "These are people I got to know because of the relationships that I built with athletics and the coach," she said.

When the YWCA honored Summitt with a lifetime achievement award in 2009, Thomas presented the pin at the ceremony. The next year in 2010, Thomas was honored with a YWCA Chrysalis award, which recognizes exemplary women in leadership positions. Summitt was invited to present the award as a surprise to Thomas. "She came from behind the curtain," Thomas said. "It was powerful." Summitt was in pain that day, as she was most days, because of her arthritic knees. Thomas was a witness to how much pain Summitt endured and how she pushed through it. "I think there are a lot of times she pushed through when she was in a lot of pain. She pushed through and had a great attitude. The amount of perseverance she showed was just incredible."

Before one game, Summitt needed to speak to a gathering of important guests at the upper reaches of Thompson-Boling Arena. Summitt and Thomas took the elevator as far as it would go and then completed the trek by stairs. Summitt was climbing on those bad knees, and Thomas was weighed down by full police gear. "We get to the top and she's grabbing for the door and I said, 'Coach, wait!' I said, 'We both need to get ourselves together here.' She said, 'Oh, yeah, you're right.'" Summitt took a deep breath and was ready to go but Thomas asked for more time and noted, "I have all this stuff on." Summitt smiled and acknowledged that Thomas had dragged her up the stairs. And then, "she popped in there like the superstar she is."

Summitt relied on Thomas to take care of her players and sometimes be a sounding board for the coach. It was clear she respected the police officer and former basketball player. "Before one game, the team was doing horrible. It was just a bad game," said Thomas, who was waiting at halftime with the coach to return to the court. "We're standing there and she's looking out there and says, 'What do you think?' I said, 'We probably need to be rebounding and stay out of foul trouble.' She said, 'I agree. By the way, do you still have any eligibility left?' I thought that was pretty funny. And she looked at me like, 'And?' She always asked what I thought about things. You could look at her and think iconic but when you talk to her, it's like the girl next door."

Thomas, whose mother is a retired educator, stayed committed to completing her degree. She accompanied players to study hall in the 2012–13 season, her last one at Tennessee, and Summitt reminded her that she had to keep the 100 percent graduation rate intact. "She actually said it," Thomas said. On a bus ride during Summitt's last season, Thomas, who worked 12-hour police shifts in addition to being a student, was looking forward to the rest. "I hear Coach call my name," Thomas said. Summitt, who was doing cognitive tests and puzzles, wanted to inspect Thomas' iPad and compare it to hers. She wasn't impressed with the racing games loaded on Thomas' device. "Mine's better," Summitt said, laughing.

"It was a lot of fun. Even though it was busy, I had a lot of fun," Thomas said. "Coach was very open about me coming in to watch film. I was like, 'Are you serious?' I wished now I had. I don't think it's about the film as much as it's about leadership. It was amazing how open she was to say, 'You're a part of the family. Come in.'" Summitt did the same with the media at times. She knew that the better informed reporters were about her team, the better stories they could write. She periodically invited beat reporters into a scouting report film session so they would see beforehand what her team wanted to do on both sides of the ball.

While the team was on the road in Summitt's final season, Thomas always went to Summitt's hotel room and escorted her to the bus. Summitt asked each time how she looked. "I told her everything looked snappy," Thomas said. "One time we were on the elevator and her collar (was slightly askew). She said, 'You can't let me go out there looking any kind of way.' She had such realness about her."

Thomas is very familiar with dementia. She took care of her grandmother, who had the illness, for years. Thomas stayed in touch with Summitt through frequent text messages. In August 2014, Thomas sent a text and the phone rang. It was Summitt. "She was just as bright as ever," Thomas said. "For a girl like me who grew up in South Georgia . . . and somehow my life makes a turn and I am walking next to her."

24

THE LADY VOL INVITATIONAL

The 2012 SEC Tournament was held in Nashville, just 52 miles from Pat Summitt's hometown of Henrietta. If it was to be her final conference tourney, there could be no better location. No matter where the SEC held its postseason shindig, the Lady Vol fans would turn it orange and white. That was the case at other venues in Duluth, Georgia, and Little Rock, Arkansas, and Nashville especially would be no different.

Summitt had famously said that without Tennessee, the conference tourney could be played in a high school gym. And she was correct. When she made those remarks, it was both a salute to the Lady Vol fans and a reaction to the league's consideration of moving the event to rather far-flung locations. Summitt's point was if the SEC wanted a well-attended and successful tourney, especially as far as ticket sales were concerned, the league should make the trip relatively accessible for Lady Vol fans. Duluth and Nashville made the most sense with the occasional trip west to Little Rock. Despite the 525-mile distance from Knoxville to Little Rock, Tennessee fans took over the venue. Arena personnel, while maintaining neutrality publicly, privately cheered for Tennessee. If the Lady Vols didn't make it to the title game, the arena, restaurants, and downtown hotels would take a significant financial hit because of fan departure.

I would joke that when the Lady Vols won a game in the SEC tourney, the loudest cheers came from the hotels, restaurants, and arena officials. Fortunately, Tennessee is often there for the final matchup. Of the 37 SEC championship games through 2016, the Lady Vols played in 23 of them and claimed 17 trophies. However, even when Tennessee departed too soon, orange-clad fans still showed up for the final game despite the absence of the Lady Vols. Rival fans and national commentators have noted their dedication to women's basketball. During the early round games, Lady Vol fans made up the largest contingent in attendance despite the fact that Tennessee was not even playing that day.

For the 2012 edition of the Lady Vol Invitational, as it was sometimes called, Tennessee entered as the No. 2 seed and thus had a first round bye as a top four seed. Tennessee practiced in the days before the March 2 game not knowing who the opponent would be as the Lady Vols geared up to face the winner of Mississippi State-Vanderbilt, but they were motivated to play either team. Vandy had poured in 93 points versus Tennessee in the regular season rematch in February, and the coaches had watched another slow start—and went quickly to the bench—in the game against Mississippi State. "Hopefully, we are going to be focused," Summitt said in a pre-tournament conference call with reporters. "Obviously, this is tough tournament, but I think our team has had some good focus and hopefully we'll come in ready to play."

Tennessee entered the tournament with four conference losses after sweeping the league in 2011, an indicator of the competitive balance of the SEC. "You've got to think Kentucky is going to be really strong," Summitt said of the tourney's No. 1 seed. "But across the board I think teams are very competitive, and it's going to be a great tournament. Every time you go out you'd better be ready to play. And if you're not you're going to go home. We want to stay in this tournament." When Nashville hosted the women's and men's tourney in the same year, it was turned orange one week by the Lady Vols, followed by Kentucky blue a week later as Wildcat fans descended on the capital of Tennessee.

During the women's tourney, because the SEC was such a deep league in terms of talent, the early round games could be very entertaining. The 2012 edition was the last year that 12 teams participated in the four-day event. In 2013, Texas A&M and Missouri joined the SEC, and the event spanned five days. The conference tourney is a fan-favorite event with multiple afternoons and evenings of basketball games. Located in the heart of downtown Nashville, Bridgestone Arena meant easy access to hotels, restaurants, and tourist attractions. The SEC member schools get first access to choice seating sections, and Lady Vol supporters often called those schools to buy prime seats for the event. Some Lady Vol fans even became season ticketholders at other SEC schools so they would have access to premium seats at tournament time. Orange-clad fans were literally seated throughout the arena.

It was fitting that the 2012 tournament was wide open in terms of which team would leave with the trophy. The Lady Vols had secured it the past two years in 2010 and 2011, but they weren't the favorites in Nashville. That distinction belonged to Kentucky as the No. 1 seed, but the Wildcats were vulnerable, as evidenced by getting waylaid in Knoxville. Nashville is Vanderbilt's hometown, but it's not the Commodores' home court since the tourney is played at Bridgestone Arena. Vandy would have its share of supporters, but Coach Melanie Balcomb knew several teams had the shot to get to Sunday's title game and win. "I've been in the conference 10 years and a lot of time teams with a bye have a huge advantage and there hasn't been that many upsets," Balcomb said. "But this year you can kind of throw out the seeds and throw out the records. When you have Alabama, a team that was on the bottom, beating Kentucky, a team that was on the top, in February that means anybody can beat anybody on a given day and there's been no rhyme or reason for a lot of things that you've seen. I definitely think in my 10 years here it's the most open tournament."

Kentucky Coach Matthew Mitchell has always enjoyed the SEC tourney and would likely attend as a fan if he were not coaching in it. "The SEC Tournament, to me, is one of the most special times of the year," Mitchell said. "I love the SEC Tournament. I think it is one of the toughest championships to win. I think it takes a herculean effort. I do think it's a wide-open tournament. I don't think that we are an unbeatable team by any stretch of the imagination. Having said that I also think that we have a team that can beat anybody in the tournament." Kentucky survived Florida in its opening game—the No. 8 seed Gators fell by four points to the Wildcats—and then got ousted by No. 4 seed LSU in the semifinals.

No. 6 seed South Carolina delivered the tournament's first upset by taking out No. 3 seed Georgia in the quarterfinals. Television commentator Van Chancellor, who had been a successful coach in the SEC and WNBA, had picked Georgia to win. Immediately after the game, South Carolina Coach Dawn Staley scooted over to the sideline and asked Chancellor: "You picked

Georgia? You picked Georgia?! You went against a point guard?!" Chancellor smiled and shook the former Olympian point guard's hand before Staley darted back to her team's celebration.

The SEC tourney is always a festive event with mascots and bands in attendance. Whenever an opposing player went to the free throw line, the Arkansas band members sang, "You're not going to make it, no you're not going to make it, you're not going to make it after all." Makes brought groans. Misses brought cheers. When it was noted that Ole Miss didn't bring its mascot, which is now a black bear, one media type on press row said: "It's still hibernating." The nickname of Ole Miss remains the Rebels, but the mascot recently had changed to a bear from Colonel Reb.

The Lady Vols' all-senior starting lineup deployed in the regular season finale in Knoxville had unleashed energy from the opening tip, and it was expected to reappear in Nashville. "They left this court and won their last game on Pat Summitt's floor," Holly Warlick said before the team departed Knoxville. "Any win for them is a boost and to go out like that was huge." When Glory Johnson was asked about Briana Bass joining the starting lineup, a huge smile broke across her face. "We seniors want to be out there together. We want to play together. We want to show people we can make a statement."

The Lady Vols always use various combinations in practice to get ready for game situations, and the five seniors had been slipping onto the practice court together in drills to send the hint that perhaps the veteran lineup would work. "We try to run out there and get ready," Johnson said. The very finite amount of time left in their careers was another factor: by putting the responsibility of a great start on the seniors, the staff hoped it was a challenge they would embrace. "Willingly we'll take that," Johnson said. "I love the responsibility."

The seniors had another team trait that was helpful: they could correct each other without causing tension. "I love holding my own seniors accountable because I grew up with them," Johnson said. "(Yell) and they'll take it the right way." The seniors also followed the scouting report on both ends against Florida, and that hadn't always happened at all five spots on the floor to start games, much to Summitt's dismay. "We had seven, eight, nine passes before someone shot the ball," Manning said. "We were very unselfish." The coaches also wanted to tap into the seniors' sense of urgency. Players in their final year can be jolted by the realization that postseason is it for them.

The Lady Vol coaching staff had a keen interest in the March 1, 2012, game between No. 7 seed Vanderbilt and No. 10 seed Mississippi State since Tennessee played the winner. A Mississippi State cheerleader did the best lobbying when she walked over to a section of Tennessee fans and asked them to cheer for the Lady Bulldogs. That group of Lady Vol fans was happy to oblige and pull against Vanderbilt. The orange-clad fans cheering for Vandy seemed eager for a rematch.

Vandy made it to the quarterfinals with a 67–51 win over Mississippi State. The game was also significant because Sharon Fanning-Otis, a long-time colleague and friend of Summitt's, coached her last game at Mississippi State, as she had announced her retirement the month prior. It also was the 400th career win for Balcomb, whose response when asked what the milestone meant was, to much laughter, "That I'm old. Sharon Fanning is leaving so now I'm the third oldest. All people are talking about is that I'm the third oldest in the SEC. It sounds like I coached a lot of games. But I don't get those wins. I don't get to play. I wasn't a real good player. Don't tell my players that."

In-state rivals Tennessee and Vanderbilt would now meet in the quarter-finals for the first time since 1991. The two teams often crossed paths in the SEC tourney, but it was usually later, in the semis or title game. Tennessee also had the element of revenge—or at least redemption—motivating them for Friday's opening game. The Commodores had poured in 93 points against Tennessee three weeks previously in the regular season matchup in Nashville. "There are a lot of things each game where we have something to prove," Warlick said. "We are not coming in as a dominant team. If that's what they want to be in this tournament then they've got to bring it. If it's a revenge factor, if it's a pride factor, whatever gets them motivated, then that is what they need to use."

Before the team left Knoxville, former Lady Vol Shelley Sexton Collier gathered the players in a circle after practice and spoke to them while they sat on the court without the Lady Vol coaches being present. Sexton Collier, the girls' basketball coach at Webb School of Knoxville, was on the first Tennessee team to win a national title in 1987. She also coached Johnson in high school. "She said she was going to make it a point to make sure she said something to us so she wouldn't regret it afterwards," Johnson said. Sexton Collier knew losses could cause some erosion of support—with the exception of the crowds at Thompson-Boling Arena all season—and she wanted the players to know she remained in their corner. Sexton-Collier had a basic message to deliver: "It's not over. The season is not over," Johnson said. "We've made mistakes. We've lost games, and we're not doing the little things. And she knows it's the Tennessee Way. It's going to take defense and rebounding."

The speech held Johnson's attention. "She was just trying to inspire us and motivate us and keep working hard for Pat. She got a little emotional when she started talking about Pat because she knows Pat. She was there with Pat when she was completely OK, and now she's dealing with it. It's a lot harder for her to watch so she decided to come say something to us. It's her trying to keep us as strong as she is. I hope it motivated other people because it motivated me. Yes, she's my high school coach, but she's watching. She's a coach. She's a former Lady Vol. She has experience. She knows how Pat is. She's played, and she's won a championship."

The SEC ran promotional announcements for Pat Summitt's foundation to raise awareness for Alzheimer's throughout the tourney. During the evening session when Tennessee was playing, the ad ran and ended with: We Back Pat. Do you?"

A Tennessee fan loudly replied: "YES WE DO!"

The players' answer needed to come on the court.

Tennessee used its senior lineup and led 13–8 before the first substitute arrived—Cierra Burdick replaced Stricklen, who had two fouls—and 15–8 before the second one did when Ariel Massengale relieved Bass. With Vicki Baugh controlling the glass for Tennessee, the Lady Vols built a 30–13 lead over Vandy with 4:20 left. But then the fouls began to pile up as Johnson and Baugh joined Stricklen on the bench with two each, and Vandy got back in the game at the free throw line.

Tennessee's lead had dwindled to eight points, 35–27, at halftime, and after a break extended by 29 minutes because severe weather needed to pass over the arena and downtown area, the Lady Vols opened the second half with four turnovers in five possessions—a Stricklen layup was the exception—and then Stricklen headed back to the bench with her third foul at the 16:14 mark. "I was really frustrated," Stricklen said. "I didn't get to play in the first half because I had two fouls. I picked up the third, got really frustrated. Coach came over there, went off on me, made it worse. I really got mad. I really felt bad because I let my teammates down."

Stricklen was sitting on the bench when the head coach leveled the senior with her stare. Stricklen responded in the second half with 18 points and a three ball that she connected after launching it from somewhere on Music Row. She reentered the game with 10:42 to play and took it over. She buried a long three to give Tennessee a 48–44 lead and then scored on an and-one play. Johnson followed that with a turn-around shot on an assist from Stricklen, plus the foul, and converted for a 54–46 lead. Stricklen buried another long three and after an errant shot by a teammate caromed off the backboard, Johnson stuck the putback for a 59–51 lead. Baugh found Stricklen for a layup in transition and a 61–53 lead and then Stricklen launched a 26-footer with one second on the shot clock that settled neatly through the net for a 64–55 lead after Kamiko Williams saved a loose ball and got it to the senior. Stricklen and Johnson sealed the 68–57 win from the line with free throws.

Stricklen may have gotten Summitt's patented stare during the game, but the head coach wrapped the senior in a huge hug afterwards. Stricklen said the Summitt stare got her going when she retook the court and that she missed the withering looks when she didn't get them.

The Lady Vols earned the right to play South Carolina in a second revenge game after the Gamecocks' takedown of Georgia. "I think we have some confidence," Staley said after South Carolina's win. "I think it's a neutral site. Tennessee played a tough game today. We played a tough game today."

Nashville had been anything but neutral—Balcomb drew laughter when she repeated a reporter's question about it being "a little tilted" to Tennessee fans—but the Gamecocks could claim the win in Knoxville. "The fact we did beat them on their floor does help with our confidence level," Staley said. Vandy was able to twice cut the lead to one point, but the Lady Vols never lost it. "This is a frustrating finish for us," Balcomb said. "We had every opportunity down the stretch. We fought hard, made good adjustments, just didn't make the plays."

Tennessee had a hand in that with its defense. "We switched around," Mickie DeMoss said. "We ran some 3–2. Sometimes we overloaded the top from the free throw line. And we ran some 2–3. The zone was pretty good to us overall. They started getting it inside in that post area. We would go zone then we would go man for a while. That bothered them a little bit. We switched off screens. We knew Melanie would adjust to whatever defense we were running. That's why we kept switching. Whatever we were running, she'd adjust. It was a well-played game, a well-coached game. It was great for our fans."

The Lady Vols and the Commodores were a few seconds away from tipping off the second half when the players and staffs were sent back to the locker room for safety reasons as tornado warnings roared across Nashville. During the 29-minute delay, hail and rain pounded the roof of Bridgestone Arena. The storm left the roof intact at Bridgestone Arena, though considerable damage occurred across the region, so the Tennessee fans did their best storm impersonation in the second half and raised enough ruckus to nearly lift it off themselves. The crowd numbered 8,594, but it sounded twice as loud and thundered to its feet in the second half behind Stricklen's sharpshooting. When Stricklen hit a three ball with 3:06 remaining that stretched a tenuous six-point lead to nine, it sounded as if another storm rumbled overhead. When asked what Stricklen's range was, Meighan Simmons smiled and said, "To half court. She practices that. It becomes fluid to her."

Halftime had been extended nearly 30 minutes past the usual 15 minutes so that the teams could hunker down in their locker rooms. Vanderbilt weathered that delay better than Tennessee as the Lady Vols turned loose of the ball to start the second half, but got back on track and, more importantly, never lost the lead. "At the beginning of the second half when we had the delay, I wasn't really pleased with how we came out," Warlick said. "It's kind of weird because we've been in a game called off at Ole Miss because of the rain, the lights went out in St. Thomas, so now we have a tornado watch. I don't know what we're doing, but. . . ." The other two weather-related incidents happened in the 2010–11 season with a power outage in the Virgin Islands and then torrential rain that blew in via the air vents at Ole Miss. It wasn't the first tornado delay for Meighan Simmons, who is from Texas. "But it wasn't as bad as this," Simmons said.

The players used the extra time to stretch, discuss the game plan, and eat some snacks. They got restless at halftime but kept stretching and moving around the confined space. "We were able to talk a little bit more about what went wrong. Holly and I were watching film a little bit," Johnson said. In a first for Baugh, extra time to rest was not what her knee needed. "I really didn't like that," Baugh said. "I've been through knee injuries. I wanted to get back and stay warm. That didn't help me and Kamiko, but the rest of them were fine." It was also a first for Johnson. "It was kind of scary," Johnson said. "They had us all secure in the locker room, but my family is out there so I was like, 'OK, if anything happens, if I hear that the roof is flying off, I am sprinting out there to go get my family.'" If Johnson had headed to the door the way she crashes the glass for rebounds, it is likely that nobody on the staff would have tried to stop her.

Postseason may seem like an odd time to make major changes to the starting lineup, but it worked as Johnson and the four other seniors worked in unison on both ends of the court. "That's probably our best defensive team," Warlick said. Surprisingly, the matchup zone worked against a team full of three-ball shooters. Typically, the way to get a team out of a defensive zone is to launch three balls over it and force tighter coverage. In the last game against Vanderbilt, Tennessee had played a mix of man and zone, and neither worked well. In the rematch in Nashville, the zone was efficient for the first half and then in the second half, the Lady Vols switched into man and back to zone at times. On Vandy's last possession, Johnson smothered Christina Foggie, and she darted left and then right before switching directions because she had no path. Vandy got a three-ball attempt from Kady Schrann but it was off, and Baugh snared the rebound to snuff the final threat. "They understand the value of defensive rebounding," Warlick said.

One of the most noticeable differences in Tennessee's defense that game was the chatter. The seniors talked constantly, and when someone missed an assignment, that player heard about it. When the underclassmen entered the game, the tone and tenor had already been set. "If they play the way they've played and continue to play, we're in good shape," Warlick said. Vandy ran an in-bounds play in the first half that bunched all four players at the elbow—the corner of the free throw line. Briana Bass had staked out her spot to defend it and was getting shoved aside by Vandy's posts. Bass dug in and didn't budge, much to the delight of the crowd as the 5'2" sparkplug held her ground against much bigger players, including the 6'4" Stephanie Holzer. "Oh, I was so mad at that big girl," Bass said. "Because I had the position first and, of course, she thought she was the bigger body, and she was going to push me out of the way. The only reason I moved is because the referee told me that I needed to be on the outside or the inside. Other than that I wasn't going to move. I was so mad."

The freshmen got their first postseason experience and acquitted themselves well. At one point in the first half, because of foul trouble for the veterans, all three freshmen were on the floor together. "I am proud of these seniors," Burdick said. "I feel like when they are playing with energy and they are playing together, they can beat any five on the floor." The Lady Vol coaches had no doubt at this point about leaving the all-senior starting lineup in place. But to reach the championship game, the Lady Vols first had to get past a pesky South Carolina team that liked to take threes and apply pressure to the ball handler.

South Carolina had a two-point lead, 11–9, at the 11:23 mark after a three-pointer from Tina Roy. Johnson got a feed from Baugh and tied the game at the rim at the 11:07 mark, and Massengale, who entered at the 13:18 mark, got a defensive board and motored to the other end for a layup and a 13–11 lead at the 10:26 mark. Tennessee did not lose the lead, but the Gamecocks stayed close and trailed by just six points, 28–22, at halftime. Stricklen arrived right on cue for the second half, and Johnson went to work inside. "She turns on at the right time," Johnson said. "I have faith in her."

The lead extended to nine points, 39–30, on a nice step-through move from Alicia Manning at the 16:23 mark of the second half. "I do think she probably settles in better when she starts," Mickie DeMoss said. "I think the seniors realize that time is running out a little bit. A-Town's focus, to me, is a little bit keener than it was, say, midseason."

Manning had a game highlight when Taber Spani curled to the paint, and Manning, who was near the top of the floor, saw the play developing. Spani converted at the rim for a 69–48 lead with 3:41 left in the game. "It was a great pass by A-Town," Spani said. Manning laughed when asked how peeved she would have been if Spani had missed the layup after a perfect feed. Manning heard directions to pull out the ball, but she saw Spani and had to turn loose. "She was working too hard so I had to let it go," Manning said. "I have faith in her."

Tennessee secured a 74–58 win in a semifinal game that stayed close until the final nine minutes when the Lady Vols got a double-digit lead—the result of an aggressive man defense—and never surrendered it. That came about by two blocks, one from Stricklen with the shot clock about to expire and an emphatic swat from Baugh. Both led to run-outs by the Lady Vols and back-to-back baskets from Massengale and Johnson. "It's a momentum builder. It's a transition basket. That's what we want," Warlick said.

South Carolina had stayed within single digits of Tennessee until the back-to-back blocks, and then Stricklen and Johnson went to work. They scored inside and out, and a game that had been within reach for the Gamecocks was suddenly effectively over. After the final missed shot by South Carolina, Massengale got the ball and dribbled out the clock. Massengale was still dribbling near the scorer's table for the final two seconds when Summitt and Staley shook hands. The crowd of 11,029—nearly 90 percent Tennessee fans—roared its approval of the outcome. "Our fans are just absolutely incredible," Warlick said. "I never thought I would say this, that the arena would sound like Thompson-Boling. But that was a loud crowd, and we're so appreciative of them coming out and supporting us. It's a tribute to this team, to Coach Summitt. I'm just proud to be from Tennessee and know how many people we have that love our basketball team."

Staley noted the talent and senior experience of Tennessee and said after the game, "I hope they get Coach Summitt another SEC Championship." Staley was also a Johnson fan, it seemed. Four seniors led the Gamecocks, but with the game out of reach in the latter part of the second half, Staley inserted underclassmen to give them some experience. "We did try to put a team of five out there that would play in this situation next year just to give them a little experience at it, to play against a team like Tennessee, playing against Glory Johnson," Staley said.

Summitt had to get Stricklen in gear again and switched approaches with a friendly chat on the baseline before the second half started. It worked again, as Stricklen erupted for 16 points, all in the second half. It was suggested that Summitt should just confront Stricklen at the pre-game meal before the title game and get a head start. That suggestion brought smiles from the Lady Vols, including Stricklen, but it would bring a bigger smile to Summitt if her senior All-American would get going in the first half. Before the second half started, Summitt spoke calmly to Stricklen on the baseline, smiling and staying positive, and that worked, too. That Summitt can reach Stricklen was apparent. She had done so for the senior's four years at Tennessee. But a faster start for Stricklen would benefit the Lady Vols to say the least.

The good news for Tennessee was that it could weather the delay for Hurricane Kinna to arrive. With Baugh and Johnson holding down the inside, Manning hitting enough shots to make the defense account for her, and the bench players providing some instant offense, Tennessee was getting team-wide contributions. It also helped that Stricklen hit a layup 10 seconds into the second half and then drained a three-pointer two minutes later on a pass from Manning. That was followed by a steal from Bass and then a Johnson finish at the rim. In between Stricklen's buckets was a Baugh spin move to the basket. In less than three minutes, all five seniors had contributed to the offensive output in some way by working in sync. It was a live game example for the underclassmen, and it's something these seniors didn't get when they arrived because of graduation and injuries that forced so many of them onto the court before they were ready for the responsibility.

It was likely an adjustment for the underclassmen who were used to starting or logging a lot of minutes, but their day was coming. Massengale was still playing considerable minutes and that would continue. Burdick saw her minutes trimmed, but based on the way she celebrated with her teammates in the locker room, she embraced her role and this team. Harrison knew she was playing behind senior posts and would become a primary post piece as a sophomore. Junior Kamiko Williams was coming back from knee surgery and made the most of her minutes, even keeping her point guard skills handy. Spani was physically limited by her knee but logged an effective nine minutes, all in the second half. Sophomore Meighan Simmons logged all of her nine minutes in the first half. She didn't play in the second, because the combination of players on the floor was working.

"That group was going well and sometimes players have to understand that that's part of the gig that when another group is going well, you may not get back in the game or get the minutes that you normally get," Dean Lockwood said. Simmons, like all of the reserves, had to stay ready and prepare as if they could play at any time. If the bench needed an example of why, all they needed to do was look at the seniors. Only Johnson and Stricklen had been regular starters, but when Bass, Manning, and Baugh were summoned to seize control of the team, they were prepared to do it.

Coupled with LSU's win over Kentucky in the other semifinal, the title game restored the natural order of the SEC universe as the Lady Vols and Tigers renewed their postseason battles. Warlick said she would change one thing by not chatting with her close friend, LSU Coach Nikki Caldwell, who is a former Lady Vol player and assistant coach. "We talk before each game," Warlick said. "It's going to be different because I'm not calling her. As much as I love Nikki Caldwell, she's not going to be a great friend of mine (on game day). Maybe after the game."

The semifinals provided some entertaining moments, especially the sight of a very pregnant Caldwell berating the officials during LSU's game against Kentucky. Press row members openly wondered if she would go into labor two weeks before the due date, as Caldwell looked ready to pop. The best media quip was: "How long would that delay halftime?" Caldwell's contractions began on the team bus after that Sunday's championship game, and she gave birth just two days later on March 6, 2012, to Justice Simone Fargas, her daughter with former NFL player Justin Fargas, Caldwell's then fiancé who is now her husband. A native of Oak Ridge, Tennessee, with a rich Lady Vols history, Caldwell was a crowd favorite in Nashville. When she gave the officials an earful, standing back because of the baby bump, fans erupted, and when an LSU player was called for a charge, an aghast Caldwell yelled, "Flop! Flop! Flop!"

The crowd also cheered whenever Summitt informed the officials what she thought about some of their calls. When Summitt stood up, lowered her eyes at the officials and then threw her arms up in the air, the orange-clad fans roared. The SEC tourney is a very media-accessible event with the locker rooms open for interviews after the games. The Lady Vols' post-game snacks were nutritious and featured apples and little cups of peanut butter for dipping. Of course, that can make video and TV interviews a little tricky as the players scrambled to wipe mouths clean, get peanut butter off their teeth and drink something to clear their throats. "Stop eating!" is the order yelled out when the media entered the locker room, but it didn't always work. The food was in front of them, and the players were hungry.

Interviewing players in their natural habitat also revealed their quirky and humorous sides. Burdick and Baugh tried to get different media members to note that the other was a loser in what appeared to be a running joke. When answering a serious question about player roles, Baugh responded and then added, "especially this loser, Cierra." Baugh reacted with mock indignation when told that Burdick had said the same thing about her. "Oh, no she didn't!" Baugh said. "She's the biggest loser. We have to love her because she's on the team and she's a great basketball player, but besides that, she's a loser. I tried to befriend her because I feel bad for her." Burdick was within earshot and whistled a peanut at Baugh's head with help from a teammate. "Sorry, they're immature," Baugh said.

Strength and Conditioning Coach Heather Mason departed ahead of the team to start getting the ice tubs ready for the players back at the hotel. Stricklen, who used to dread the cold dips, now looked forward to them because of the relief it provided to her legs. Johnson didn't like them, but she knew the benefits so she took the icy plunge. Baugh apparently despised them, and Johnson said her post mate might slip a little hot water into the tub to make it bearable. "Oh, that is not true," Baugh said. "I get in the ice bath. It takes me a long time to get in there because it hurts, but after the first minute you're fine." Tennessee would be playing three tough and physical games in three days, so a deep freeze was vital. "Eat a lot, ice baths, and go to bed early," Manning said.

A physical player, Johnson had just one foul called against South Carolina, and she was thrilled. "That one was a foul," Johnson agreed. "That was correct. I did foul her in help side (defense)." Of course, the flip side was that Johnson rarely heard whistles for all the fouls she absorbed. She had one South Carolina player repeatedly dig into the back of her legs and try to steer her out of the paint. On one play, the defender had nearly ridden Johnson out to the arc, where the official had finally seen enough and called it. "I would be posting up, and she would be underneath me," Johnson said. Johnson took another physical pounding but maintained her composure. "I try talking to the refs; if it doesn't happen I try talking to Dean," Johnson said, referring to Dean Lockwood. "Dean keeps me composed. He keeps me calm. If I relax, my coaches will take care of it. It happens from the beginning of the game to the end."

Although she left in 2008 to become the head coach at UCLA before the seniors arrived on campus, Caldwell had helped to recruit this senior class for Tennessee, so she knew them well. Caldwell was also as steeped in Lady Vol lore as anyone else in Nashville was that weekend. But in the

SEC title game, she would be trying to lead her Lady Tigers to a win over Tennessee. "Nikki knows us like the back of her hand," Manning said. "It's really going to be a game of execution and hard work and passion."

"It's going to be a fight," Baugh said. "And we have to be mature and composed." Caldwell's team played like one coached by Summitt, and the Lady Vols had noticed. "We're playing ourselves," Baugh said. "I am looking forward to a really physical game, and it's going to be a game for big kids. I just wish her all the best, but we're going to have to kick her butt."

25

SEC TOURNAMENT CHAMPIONSHIP

The game began with a group hug among Tennessee's Pat Summitt, Holly Warlick, and Mickie DeMoss and LSU's Nikki Caldwell and Tasha Butts, who also played for Tennessee. And then, as often happens when these two teams meet, a battle ensued.

LSU opened the game in a matchup zone as the Lady Tigers had done throughout the tourney with teams struggling to get inside and find open shots. Tennessee moved the ball around on its first possession and got it to Vicki Baugh near the free throw line, but she was swarmed and passed to Glory Johnson with the orders to shoot because the shot clock was about to expire. Johnson, however, was at the arc. She missed two three-ball shots as a freshman, hit her only attempt as a sophomore—a highlight-reel toss that she had to fling sideways as the shot clock expired—and didn't even try one as a junior. But Johnson somehow drained her first attempt as a senior 38 seconds into the game with the shot clock at one on a busted play, much to the delight of the crowd. Johnson, who noted where her feet were, gathered herself for a split second right before she released the ball. "I held my follow-through," Johnson said, using the same shooting technique that Dean Lockwood drilled into her for four seasons with her midrange game. "I realized that I was at the three-point line and said, 'OK, let me hold my follow-through as long as I can, so it's not short.'"

The 3–0 lead, of course, didn't last long as Jones hit a layup for LSU followed by a tip-in from Adrienne Webb. Manning tied the game for Tennessee with a trey at the 15:45 mark of the first half, her third three-pointer of the tourney on five attempts. LSU got the lead back on a layup by Theresa Plaisance and then Tennessee went up three, 15–12, after a three ball from Briana Bass and two layups from Baugh, including a spin move to the basket with 12:03 left in the first half. LSU led twice more, 16–15 and then 23–22, before Tennessee took the lead, 25–23, on a three from Taber Spani at the 5:09 mark, but the Tigers hovered throughout the half. Tennessee stretched the lead to seven points, 32–25, after Johnson made four consecutive free throws, but LSU cut the lead to 33–30 after two free throws by LaSondra Barrett. Shekinna Stricklen found Isabelle Harrison inside for a layup and a 35–30 lead with 53 seconds left before halftime, and that completed the scoring in the first 20 minutes. Every basket was earned.

LSU pushed the Lady Vols throughout the second half. "I think when our back is against the wall, these ladies had a toughness that we haven't had in a long time," Warlick said. "It showed in the three games that we played." The Lady Tigers were able to tie the game at 41 within five minutes of the second half, but Stricklen got the lead back with two free throws. On Tennessee's next possession a Massengale pass intended for Johnson got tipped away, but an alert Baugh grabbed it and finished at the rim for a 45–41 lead.

On LSU's next possession, Barrett missed a jumper and went down in traffic in the paint. As Manning, who got the rebound, and Johnson turned up court, Barrett went to get up and caught a knee from Johnson to her head. Barrett was removed on a stretcher after a delay for treatment, and she waved to the relieved crowd as she was wheeled off before being taken to a local hospital. "I tried to avoid it," Johnson said. "I didn't think she was going to lift up her head as soon as she did. She caught the side of my leg. A-Town went that way, and I went this way. She's a great player and she's an awesome person off the court. We still keep in touch, and I will make sure that I check on her later." After diagnostic tests that included a CT scan, it was determined that Barrett had a concussion, and she was released to travel home with the team. "We could have easily folded after LaSondra went down," Webb said. "But we took it as a challenge, to not go out there and quit, but give it our all, put our hearts into the game."

LSU trimmed the lead to one point, 45–44, on a three from Webb, but Stricklen was fouled by Jeanne Kenney on a three attempt with the shot clock about to expire and drained all three for a 48–44 lead with 12:52 left. Stricklen stuck a baseline shot with one second on the shot clock for a 50–44 lead and followed that with another baseline shot for a 52–44 lead with 10:49 left. "I think she turns on when she needs to turn on," Johnson said. "She knows that she has to help our team win, and that is what she does. She hits big shots whether it's deep threes or crashing the boards with me."

LSU still had fight left and cut the lead to 56–51 on a Webb layup with 5:13 to play, but Tennessee kept finding answers from Massengale's free throws to Johnson's inside play to Stricklen's two clutch shots. "These are the best games to play," Massengale said. "Top competition is going back and forth, back and forth. The blowouts, they're fun to get the win, but when it comes down to it we want to play good basketball." When LSU brought pressure, Massengale motored through it, and Tennessee stuck the shots. LSU was forced to foul and Massengale made five of six free throws down the stretch for the final 70–58 score. Summitt told her players that this was her favorite team right before they took the court. The favored daughters then went out and won their third straight SEC Tournament title. A record championship game crowd of 12,441 showed up at Bridgestone Arena and watched the Lady Vols win their 16th SEC Tournament title in program history.

Tennessee held off a rugged LSU team in true Lady Vol tradition with defense and board play. Two blocks by Kamiko Williams with less than five minutes to play led to Tennessee points on the next possessions—a drive by Massengale and a three from Stricklen. It was a typical Tennessee-LSU game in that both teams wanted to own the paint, get to the free throw line, and control the boards. Tennessee, led by its seniors, set the tone for all three games in Nashville and departed with the trophy. "Glory Johnson, Vicki Baugh, that Shekinna are all great players," LSU's Courtney Jones said. "That's just their game, and you have to match their intensity." LSU did, and the result was another pitched battle between the storied SEC programs. "Even though the outcome didn't come out our way, much credit to the Tennessee team," Caldwell said.

The Lady Vols got the outcome they wanted by playing one of the best versions of Tennessee basketball that they had all season. "It's just an awesome feeling," Warlick said. "About two, three weeks ago we went back to work. These young ladies bought into what we needed to do." When the clock struck zero, the celebration began for the Lady Vols, their redemption in the first postseason tourney of 2012 secured. After the handshake line with the Lady Tigers—the Lady Vols hugged Destini Hughes, who shredded her knee during the game in Knoxville—Tennessee gathered at center court for the trophy presentation with SEC Commissioner Mike Slive, who saluted Summitt as the greatest coach in the game. Johnson, who had 58 points and 30 rebounds over three games, was the MVP.

Stricklen and Johnson looked at each other and got tears in their eyes as they watched Summitt climb the ladder and cut down the net at Bridgestone Arena. This was Tennessee's third consecutive SEC Tournament title, but this one was the most special, especially for the seniors. "I think we really solidified what we should have been doing in the regular season in the SEC," Manning said. It had been a trying regular season with eight losses, including three at home, but that paled compared to the announcement that roiled the team last August that their iconic head coach had been diagnosed with dementia. These seniors were also seeking their first Final Four and had at times been cited more for what they hadn't done than for what they had accomplished. So imagine Summitt telling those players minutes before tipoff that they were her favorite team. According to Stricklen, the players exploded out of the locker room.

What they encountered was a tough LSU team coached by the mirror image of Summitt in Caldwell, but as the Lady Vols had done for three games in Nashville, they got the halftime lead and they never trailed in the second half. Warlick had said she wasn't going to call or text Caldwell before the title game, but she he did anyway that Saturday night. "I texted her and I told her I hope her water broke so she wouldn't be on the court," Warlick said. "She texted me that it did, and she had a little point guard ready to play. We coach against a lot of people. But obviously Nikki is one of my best friends. So excited for us. Sorry for her."

Tennessee learned quite a bit about itself in Nashville and found a starting lineup with the five seniors. The Lady Vols also solidified roles off the bench with players settling into, and accepting, what they could bring to the court. The players joked that they also found a new three-ball threat in Johnson. "Glory is an All-American, so clearly don't leave her open," Cierra Burdick said. "Man, that shocked everybody!" Massengale added, "I think we knew when she hit that shot, that it was going to be a good day for us." Manning connected on three treys in Nashville, but she declared Johnson the better shooter. "Look at the stats, obviously Glory, 100 percent," Manning said. "She had to take it. I knew right then and there it was going to be one of those games. It was fun."

Stricklen let out a long no when asked if Johnson was now better from long range than she was. Johnson let out a long no when asked if she was a three-ball shooter now. "Only when I have to," Johnson said. "Only when the shot clock is going down and they say, 'Shoot it.' Vicki told me to shoot it. I let it go." Meanwhile, Stricklen's slow starts continued in Nashville, but the senior delivered every second half. Stricklen scored 50 points in Nashville with 48 coming after halftime. "Mickie coaches the first half; I coach the second," Warlick joked.

Williams was now entering games for her defense, a notion that would have been unheard of when she was a much-maligned underclassman because of porous defense, and she delivered with two swats to snuff out any chance of an LSU comeback. "Her defense was absolutely pivotal for us, figuratively speaking, holding the fort," Dean Lockwood said. "They were making a real run at us. The two blocks were the things that stood out, but her position defense (was big). Her ability to force Jeanne Kenney into her weak hand, making her go left rather than allowing her to go right, was huge for this team . . . and it was a big part of us winning this game."

It was Lockwood who suggested inserting Williams for defense on the bench in Nashville, and hearing the words out loud startled even him. "I remember saying it and thinking, 'What did I just say? Who said that?'" She is so capable. That kid is so understated athletically. She can guard people when she wants to. When we want to lock up on the perimeter and she's engaged, she's going to have that opportunity." An engaged Williams can be a shutdown defender, a crucial role in postseason. Williams tore the ACL in her left knee in July 2011 and rehabbed with an eye on coming back for the 2011–12 season. She was cleared to play in games in late December. "I wanted it," Williams said. "I wanted it for this team. Getting hurt kind of opened my eyes, and I am grateful to come back this year, and I am not going to take it for granted. This is my last year to play with the seniors. I busted my tail when I was hurt to play with them, so I am not going to let up."

Summitt's mantra was defense and board play, and while some may tire of hearing it, her system does work at all levels of the game. The Lady Vols got stops when they needed them and dominated LSU on the boards, 39–23. Johnson led the way with 11 rebounds. Seconds before the final horn sounded Theresa Plaisance missed a three attempt, and Johnson got the ball in a battle for it. She held on in the scrum and was credited with that final rebound as time expired. "I keep saying every game, I don't think she can take it to another level, and she keeps taking it to another level," Warlick said. "That's just her nature. She's competitive. I absolutely love that about Glory. It's in her spirit; it's in her DNA."

Lockwood coached Lady Vol legends Nicky Anosike and Candace Parker. While talking to Mickey Dearstone on the post-game radio show, Lockwood was asked if he had ever been around a player that went as hard as Johnson. "No. In one word, no," Lockwood said. "This is my 32nd year of coaching basketball. I've been around some really great competitors. Dan Majerle comes to mind at Central Michigan and some others. Male or female, Glory Johnson plays as hard and is as fiercely competitive as any player that I've had the honor of coaching."

The freshman Burdick had tremendous respect for the senior. "I am just glad she is on my team and I'll say it until I hit the grave, because if I were playing against her, I would tell my team just to put in their mouth guards because the hits are coming," Burdick said. "Glory is a workhorse. She is going to work for all 40 minutes and if we go into overtime, she is going to work for those, too. She is going for every rebound, she is hustling, she's diving and there is no player like Glory out there in the league at all." Burdick said if she ever were assigned to guard Johnson in a game, she would consider football-type gear. "I would seriously put every single pad possible on my body and just hope to God I could get a charge," Burdick said. An LSU player took a charge from Johnson in the first half and had to sit for a few seconds to gather herself before getting up. Fortunately for that player, there was a brief stop in play for substitutions. Burdick took a charge from Johnson in practice once that season. "Never again will I do that," Burdick said.

Summitt saluted Johnson's board work and that of Baugh, who grabbed seven rebounds, and Manning, who tallied six boards, with five coming in the first half to lead the team. It took nearly four years, but the Lady Vols, with the seniors leading the way, were finally playing in Summitt's image. Summitt was in her 38th year of coaching. That this was her favorite team might have seemed surprising at first, but consider how far this team, especially the seniors, traveled. "We've played well and not well," Lockwood said. "Through it all, this group stayed the course. I think it did take them awhile to embrace defense and rebounding as the pillars of really great basketball and what this program is built on. Not that they didn't believe it, but it's one thing to believe it, and it's another thing to really live it out on a daily basis."

Stricklen and Johnson had started since they were freshmen because of graduation and injuries. Both played out of position without complaint, Stricklen at point guard when needed and Johnson at center for most of her career despite having the slender body of a forward. That evening in Nashville, watching Summitt climb the ladder to snip the net was an emotional moment for both of them. Among those in attendance were Summitt's mother, Hazel Head, and her son Tyler, who had played his Senior Day game for the Vols the day before in Knoxville with a video message delivered by his mother. Pat Summitt recorded the message inside Pratt Pavilion before her team departed for the SEC tourney, and the appearance of the Lady Vols head coach on the overhead scoreboard at Thompson-Boling Arena caused the crowd in Knoxville to erupt.

"Hey, Tyler, this is Mom," Summitt said on the video. "I wish I could be there, but I am going to be in Nashville as you know. I tell everyone that you are my rock, and I love you. I want you to go out and play hard and enjoy this. I think you understand more about basketball than about anybody I know, and I know that you will leave here and become a coach. Just know that I am going to be with you always and support you always. And I love

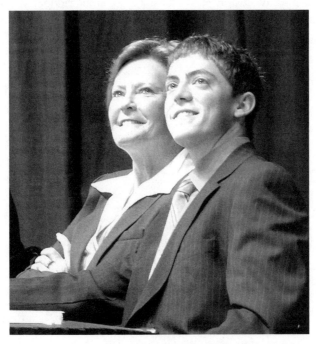

Pat Summitt and her son, Tyler Summitt, watch a photo montage during the press conference to announce her retirement.

you." When the camera went back to Tyler, who was accompanied by his father, R. B. Summitt, there were tears in his eyes.

Now, the fans in Bridgestone Arena were at full roar at the sight of Summitt on the ladder in Nashville. "We just all looked at each other and started screaming, 'Wow, she's about to cut it!'" Stricklen said. "Nobody deserves it better than our coach." The realization that it could be the last time Summitt scaled a ladder wasn't lost on the long-timers, including Debby Jennings and Meshia Thomas. "It was tough to watch, but it felt good to have her do that," Thomas said. You can't cry at that moment. You just want to soak it in."

Summitt had taken a snip from the net and was headed down the ladder when her players told her to cut it all down. So, Summitt took the scissors all over the twine. "She's got to learn to cut down nets a little better," Warlick quipped. "She chewed the net up so bad, I don't think we can put it around the trophy." Warlick had broken her hand disembarking from a plane in preseason, and DeMoss broke her arm after falling when her long untied shoelaces were stepped on during a road trip in California.

"Pat is the only healthy one that can climb up the ladder," Warlick said. "We told her to have at it."

26

PRACTICE AND REST

The Lady Vols were in a good place after the SEC postseason, in part because of what took place before it started.

The players had confided in Jenny Moshak that they were emotionally spent. Moshak made arrangements with the staff to have a psychologist talk to the team. Sports psychology is common among teams, but the Lady Vols needed help with what had happened to their head coach. "It was so much like the elephant in the room, and we were never able to get all of our feelings out," Cierra Burdick said. "Finally, they brought in a therapist for the team. That was when we were able to find a little bit of peace." The season-wide focus had been to create normalcy, but the players were frayed at that point. "We wished we had done it earlier," Burdick said. "We were doing what basketball players do. Keep going. That is our mentality. You play through pain."

The timing of the SEC postseason tournament meant the Lady Vols had two weeks before the Big Dance started. It is a break both players and coaches appreciate. After the scintillating wins in Nashville, the team had the day off before getting back to practice for three days, followed by two off days in a row. Glory Johnson traded ice baths for relaxing bubble baths at home and rested her battered body before the next round of postseason. "Outside of going to class, I will be resting my feet, elevating my feet, and taking baths," Johnson said. "That's my thing, bubble baths, relax."

Johnson also planned to take a fishing trip with Shekinna Stricken. Johnson, who is from Knoxville, is a high heels and fashion maven, while Stricklen, who is from Arkansas, considers fishing to be the best way to spend an idle afternoon. The pair made plans to head to Norris Lake to drop a line. Knowing how intense Johnson was on the court, Stricklen wasn't sure if she could switch to the laid-back style that fishing required. She wondered if Johnson had the patience for piscatorial pursuits, and had long ago concluded that Summitt would be a bad fishing partner for that very reason. Johnson said she had a little experience with baiting a hook, but she had no desire to catch any large fish. "I want the small ones, because I am not going to touch it if the fish is huge," Johnson said.

Lockwood wanted a scouting report from Stricklen about where she drops her line. "She could probably give me a real education on fishing spots around here," he said. He was surprised that Johnson agreed to bait the hook and not surprised that Stricklen, an avid angler, would handle removal of any caught fish. "Here's the paradox," Lockwood said. "Such a rough-and-tumble player, probably as physical a player as there is in the country, and she won't get near a fish."

The five seniors stood on the sideline at practice that Wednesday after their success in Nashville and smiled as they spoke to one another and pointed out action on the court. "I love it," Johnson said. "That is what we were thinking about before the senior game. We have the responsibility; we have everything on our shoulders. We can play together, and we can play strong, and we can get the job done, so let's go out there and do it."

It was the following Monday when the NCAA brackets would be announced—and the Selection Committee revealed, yet again, its tendency to be tone deaf to the women's game—so the team wasn't preparing yet for an opponent. The committee was often too populated with representatives of smaller schools, many dribbles removed from big-time college basketball. The NCAA's most important event of the year was left to those who, quite frankly, had little stake in it. Joan Cronan, a well-respected athletics director, had never served on the committee, an omission that was staggering. The process did improve—as did the overall selection process—when Dru Hancock became chair of the Division I Women's Basketball Committee, effective September 1, 2014. The senior associate commissioner of the Big 12 Conference, Hancock was a former basketball and tennis player at Ohio State, where she earned a bachelor's degree in speech communication and a master's degree in journalism. She had also served as women's associate athletics director at Tennessee. Hancock had the bona fides to oversee the sport's signature event.

Practices during that week following the SEC Tournament were more about fine-tuning some offensive and defensive strategies, working on shooting repetition, and getting some rest before the NCAA Tournament began. Recruiting, of course, never ends, especially in March when a lot of high schools across the country are playing in district and state championship playoffs. Pat Summitt, Mickie DeMoss, and Holly Warlick were on the road, so Dean Lockwood handled one session that week on his own.

Summitt and Warlick were in Georgia to see high school class of 2013 standout Diamond DeShields, who, partly due to the uncertainty of Summitt's future, chose North Carolina over several top programs, including Tennessee. She regretted her decision soon after arriving in Chapel Hill and thought about transferring immediately, but her mother told her daughter to play the 2013–14 season and reevaluate the situation after one year at North Carolina. A few weeks after the Tar Heels' season ended in the Elite Eight in March 2014, North Carolina announced that DeShields would transfer. On June 12, 2014, the national freshman of the year, without fanfare or publicity, signed her name to scholarship papers in Warlick's office.

"I feel like the lights and the cameras are for a celebration, and that is for a high school celebration," DeShields said. "You are celebrating going to college. I didn't feel like I needed to stick my chest out and be boastful with this process." Her three finalists were Tennessee, South Carolina, and Georgia, and she made visits to all three schools, but the Lady Vols emerged quickly as the front-runner, in part because DeShields had been a fan of the Lady Vols since childhood. Her decision to go to Tennessee should not have been a surprise to anyone who had been paying attention. "I had some good schools to pick from, but my vision was clear here," DeShields said. "The vision of being here actually has been a part of my entire life. I always dreamed of playing at Tennessee, and I had a very successful detour at North Carolina, but I feel like I'm back on track. I am just thankful for Holly and everybody for giving me the opportunity."

DeShields has deep orange roots in Tennessee, as her mother, Tisha Milligan DeShields, was an All-American heptathlete in 1991. "I have been a Tennessee fan since I was born," DeShields said. "I was born into it. My mom's track teammates were always there. They basically helped raise me. They ingrained my memories with orange and baby blue and Tennessee Lady Vols. Even before I knew I wanted to be a basketball player, I knew I wanted to be a Lady Volunteer. I went to a private school and every time we were out of uniform, I wore my Tennessee sweatshirt or my orange shoes or something Tennessee."

DeShields' recruitment in high school coincided with Summitt's announcement about her health. Warlick was named head coach after the season ended, and DeShields selected North Carolina less than two months later. She had cooled on the Lady Vols under an onslaught of chatter claiming the program would go into decline, and she placed a call to Warlick to tell her before making the commitment public in 2012. Some recruits don't bother with those phone calls, but DeShields made sure the other schools recruiting her were told beforehand. "I believe that God led me there for a reason," DeShields said. "I grew a lot at North Carolina. I found clarity, and I appreciate everything that North Carolina did for me. I had a great experience, but I feel like I am where I am supposed to be at this point, and I am very excited and very happy to be here with Holly."

So, while Warlick didn't reel in DeShields on that first try, she did the second time. Warlick had already proven that she could recruit. Within weeks after DeShields selected North Carolina in 2012, Warlick got a verbal commitment from Jannah Tucker in the same high school class, a top 10 recruit. The nation's No. 1 recruit in the class of 2013, Mercedes Russell, followed in November 2012, in turn followed by standout guard Jordan Reynolds. Both Russell and Reynolds are from Oregon. Tucker is from Maryland. Warlick's first signing class spanned the continent. The Lady Vols' program was here to stay.

Tisha DeShields had wisely let Diamond make her own decision, and in the summer of 2012 she hosted a Tar Heel-blue themed party for her daughter. "As a parent, I needed to support her, even though I joked with her that I was going to buy her orange briefs to wear underneath her uniform. Now, I just feel like she's in the right place. I feel like she's found her place, on 'The Summitt.'" Warlick, who turned 56 years old the week Diamond enrolled at Tennessee in 2014, got the birthday present she wanted. "She was extremely happy," Diamond said. "Before I signed, she took my hand and did an imaginary-like sign across the form. We made light of the situation. She lost me once, and she was going to make sure it wasn't going to happen again."

But on March 8, 2012, with Summitt, Warlick, and DeMoss on the recruiting trail, Lockwood was trying to get the 2011–12 team ready for the NCAA tourney before the players got two consecutive days to rest, including a Saturday, a coveted off day because there are no classes. The veteran coach, who noted the "big cat" was away, had plenty of experience keeping the proverbial mice in line. "It was good; it was fun," Lockwood said. "Sharpness, our execution, conditioning, getting a lot of shots, not losing our competitive edge," Lockwood said. Drills included rebounding and defense—"not going away from our core values," he noted—along with shot repetition. During a brief point where Lockwood noticed the "big cat's away" mentality, he reestablished control with a few sprints. "I've done this before," said Lockwood, who was a head coach at Northwood and Saginaw Valley State universities, both in Michigan. "We can play that game. It was all right. They just needed a little friendly nudge."

Cierra Burdick, a bona fide gym rat, lofted shots after practice with Lockwood. Burdick's ability to hit shots was a direct result of her willingness to get in the gym. "No question," Lockwood said. "She is a great example of the fruits of her labors paying off in games. There is no magic in this game. There's no big secret. It's like the law of the farm. If you work your farm, you are probably going to have a good crop. But, if you half work and sleep on the front porch, you're probably not going to yield a good crop."

The day before the Selection Show always feels a bit like Christmas Eve to Tennessee, and this year what would be under the tree was a complete mystery. Drawing No. 1 Baylor's bracket would be the basketball equivalent of coal. The Bears were chewing up opponents that season. After missing the Final Four in 2011, despite having the 6'8" Brittney Griner, Baylor was on a mission in 2012. On that Sunday before the Selection Show, the Lady Vols were back in Pratt Pavilion for practice and anxious to see the brackets. "No idea, none whatsoever," Lockwood said. "We're going to be all equally surprised." With eight losses, the Lady Vols could not even be certain of a two seed, though the No. 1 strength of schedule and No. 4 RPI boosted their resume. Summitt hosted the team, staff, administrators, and media at her house for a meal before the brackets were unveiled on ESPN. The assistants then headed back to campus late that evening and began to gather film of the three other teams in their first and second round sub-regional. The three assistants each took a team for scouting purposes, and that evening they had DVDs in laptops so practice plans could be formulated accordingly for the next day.

Michael Fahey, then the team's video coordinator, had been building a library of film all season from televised and online games. "It's miniscule the number of games we can't access," Lockwood said. "Holly and Mickie and

I will get together and divvy up who's scouting what." The coaches did not limit their viewing to the assigned scout. They also checked out the entire side of their bracket. Summitt, as always, watched the next opponent. "It becomes a tape marathon," Lockwood said. "My life ceases to exist." Lockwood didn't care. He wanted the season to extend as long as possible.

27

SELECTION SHOW

P at Summitt hosted the media at her home for the annual Selection Show—always serving her famous jalapeno corn—and she told those in attendance, "If you leave my home hungry, it's your fault." Longtime attendees knew one unwritten rule: don't get between the players and the food line. They loaded their plates with salad, chicken, ribs, salmon, vegetables, rolls, and corn muffins and were followed by media, staff, and administrators. The desserts, including Summitt's homemade vanilla ice cream, took up one side of the outdoor kitchen at the pool house. Everyone got fed, and there were still plenty of leftovers to fill to-go containers.

The Lady Vols finally got a destination (Chicago) and an opponent (Tennessee-Martin) and would open NCAA tourney play on March 17, 2012, at Allstate Arena in Rosemont, a suburb of the Windy City. Tennessee is the only school that has earned a bid to every NCAA Division I tourney since the event began in 1982. Tennessee had grown restless the previous week awaiting its destination, and it landed in the same region as overall No. 1 seed Baylor. The NCAA women's Selection Committee, which has been rightly criticized for its makeup of administrators without elite Division I athletics experience, had been tone deaf in the past. In 2012, it was stunningly so.

While a Final Four slot was tough in any season, Baylor's region was a roadblock to every team in the country. While Tennessee had no guarantee of beating any of the other three No. 1 seeds, the Selection Committee essentially guaranteed Tennessee would not be at the Final Four in Summitt's last season by placing the Lady Vols with Baylor, a juggernaut in 2012 that finished 40–0. Remarkably, the Lady Vols landed in Baylor's region again in 2013, marking three times in four years (2010, 2012, and 2013) that the Selection Committee placed Tennessee with Baylor during the Brittney Griner era. Louisville, however, managed to eliminate Baylor in 2013 in a game so poorly officiated—Griner was shoved and held throughout the game without fouls being called—that the NCAA, which was concerned about the exit of the No. 1 seed in that fashion, not to mention the impact on ticket sales and hotel reservations at the Final Four, used clips from the game film the following season as a tutorial for officials about how not to call a basketball game.

But in 2012, after a week devoted to both practice and rest, the Lady Vols were restless to know who they would next play in the postseason. The answer came at the end of the nearly hour-long Selection Show as Tennessee popped in as the No. 2 seed in the Des Moines Region. The first-round opponent brought as many cheers as the sight of Tennessee's name since Tennessee-Martin is where Summitt played her college ball. She jokingly agreed that she should handle that scouting report for her assistants. The other two teams in the sub-regional were DePaul and Brigham Young University.

Tennessee was the automatic qualifier after winning the SEC Tournament and joined seven other SEC teams who made the Big Dance, including Kentucky, LSU, Georgia, South Carolina, Arkansas, Vanderbilt, and Florida, another indicator of the depth and strength of the league. "It's a great conference," Vicki Baugh said. "And I am just glad to be in it because I know it makes us prepared to handle any team."

Tennessee-Martin was the automatic qualifier from the Ohio Valley Conference and averaged 81.1 points per game. One notable score that season was a 99–84 loss to Vanderbilt. The Skyhawks were a team that liked to launch the ball from the arc; in fact, they came oh-so-close to eliminating North Carolina in the first round in 2014. They were led by OVC Player of the Year Jasmine Newsome, a sophomore guard from Millington, Tennessee, who became the second-fastest player in program history to reach 1,000 career points—ahead of Summitt and behind teammate Heather Butler, a First

Team All-OVC selection, who led the team with 98 three-pointers that season. Jaclissa Haislip, a forward/guard from Murfreesboro, Tennessee, is the cousin of Marcus Haislip, who played for the Vols and was drafted into the NBA in 2002. Haislip had 65 treys on the season. As a team the Skyhawks had 323 made treys on the season. Taylor Hall, a senior guard from Mt. Juliet, Tennessee, who transferred from Roane State in 2010, had connected on 71.

Needless to say, the Lady Vols would have to guard the long ball.

Summitt, a 1974 graduate of the school in West Tennessee, began her career as head coach of the Lady Vols that same year while working on her master's degree in Knoxville. The Skyhawks had beaten Tennessee twice—in 1971 and 1972, when Summitt was on the team. The Lady Vols had won the other 13 matchups. The announcement of the site brought a shriek of joy from freshman Ariel Massengale, who is from nearby Bolingbrook, Illinois, and would play close to home in front of family and friends. "Massengale goes home so hopefully she'll bring a lot of relatives and fans," Mickie DeMoss said. "We have a lot of UT fans in the Chicago area, and I think we have fans that will travel."

Tennessee may have drawn the overall No. 1 seed in Baylor, but Des Moines, the site of the regional, was not on the minds of the Lady Vols. "Not this early," DeMoss said. "You start thinking about Baylor, you are going to get beat in the first game. You've got to have total focus on the game in hand." Junior Taber Spani nodded when asked the same question. "Absolutely," Spani said. "We're guaranteed one game so it has got to be that mindset."

Spani remained limited by the left knee injury that hindered her mobility all season. The days off were good for the knee, but she would not be well until she got extended off-season rest. Spani wanted to contribute when she could, especially for the five seniors. "That is obviously motivation and bigger motivation is doing it for Pat," Spani said. Senior Briana Bass wasn't focused as much on which teams were in the bracket as she was on how the Lady Vols would play. "There are a lot of last times of everything going on this year," she said. Indeed, Monday was Baugh's fifth, and final, Selection Show. "They are all special," Baugh said. "You don't know what you are going to get. It's fun to see where you end up. We're very excited, and we knew it was going to be tough. It always is."

Kamiko Williams had been fielding questions about Baylor, but she noted they "were way at the top" of the bracket and the Lady Vols were at the bottom of it as the two seed, and she preferred to discuss Tennessee-Martin. "I am excited for coach's sake," Williams said. "But we've just got to take it a game at a time because like Kara (Lawson) said (during the show), sometimes we've been inconsistent and when our energy is not there we have a tendency to play down to our opponent. We have seen some upsets, and anything can happen at tournament time."

The Lady Vols had to wait until the last bracket was announced to learn their destination. It made the three freshmen a tad anxious. "Rel (Ariel Massengale) was getting a little nervous," Williams said. "She didn't know where we were going to be." It gave the seniors a little more time to reflect. "About halfway through I looked at Bree and Strick and said, 'Wow, this is the last time we're going to be doing this,'" Alicia Manning said. "We're all really excited. It's kind of bittersweet, but this is our time. I love Chicago so I am excited about it."

One of the happiest players after the bracket announcement was Massengale. Her scream pierced the television viewing room in Summitt's pool house when she realized the team was headed to Chicago. "She had better bring that in Chicago," Williams said with Massengale listening nearby, laughing. "I see her over there getting excited, 'WE'RE IN CHICAGO!' If she plays like a scrub, I am talking bad about her. Put that on tape." An Arkansas native, Stricklen had hoped for Little Rock as an early round site, but she was happy for Massengale. "It feels good to let Rel go home. We know she is the homesick one on the team," Stricklen said. "It's good that she's there. She'll bring it."

Meighan Simmons watched Summitt's reaction to the bracket and saw a familiar look from her head coach, especially when Martin was paired with the Lady Vols. "I think she is going to be so ready," Simmons said. "I feel like she has got that Pat Summitt kind of mood right now. You could tell from her reaction." Summitt was indeed fired up that week, especially March 14, the day before the team departed for Chicago. Jere Longman of *The New York Times* was in town and followed Summitt and the Lady Vols throughout the NCAA postseason. On March 14, Summitt met with the media in Pratt Pavilion. The head coach was feisty when the question about her coaching future was raised. "Oh, I haven't made any decision about that," Summitt said.

The reply was notable because Summitt had met that day with Athletics Director Dave Hart, and her future had been discussed. The conversation eventually became part of a lawsuit by Debby Jennings, ultimately settled for $320,000 out of court, who asserted that Summitt had been directed to step down at the end of the season. UT administrators hovered in Pratt Pavilion that day, presumably to hear what Summitt would tell *The New York Times* and other assembled media. Summitt, as always, took the high road. She would never put such media focus on herself, especially with her team about to tip off the NCAA tourney.

Summitt was particularly animated that day, so much so that beat reporters noticed the difference and inquired about it. That familiar flash was back in her eyes. From a broader point of view, Summitt said, "I love the game. And whether I'm here at UT, I may or may not coach. It is what it is. I'm just trying to get another championship for this group." That was Summitt's focus the entire season—that team, and in particular, that senior class. Warlick noted that, to some extent, she and Summitt had shifted duties. "I think Pat and my roles almost have reversed," Warlick said. "I usually am doing a little bit more one-on-one with kids and Pat a little bit more coaching. If there's a positive with this situation, it's that Pat has had more time to spend one-on-one with our kids. It has been very powerful, and they have responded well. She is really focusing in on these kids."

Cierra Burdick was jumping rope when she was summoned for an interview. She took a break, wiped sweat off her face and smiled. Practice was already over, but the freshman figured she still had time to get better. She asked if video would be taken—no, so it was safe to pour sweat throughout the interview, which she did. "Just trying to get the feet quicker," Burdick said of her jump-rope sessions after practice. "Just trying to be able to slide with these quicker guards." It was that dedication to the game that had the coaches comfortable with bringing the freshman off the bench in postseason, even in crunch time, which was the staff's ultimate sign of trust.

Burdick's extra workouts were intended to help her on defense. The coaches did not hesitate to put her in a game for offensive reasons. "We have a lot of faith in her right now, especially if they're playing zone," Lockwood said. Tuesday had been the team's off day—the players had midterm exams that week—but Burdick was in Pratt Pavilion anyway and summoned Lockwood to help her. "Dean and I got a great workout in," Burdick said. "We got 313 makes up (jump shots), 116 made free throws. It was hardcore, a little conditioning in as well." Burdick was looking forward to spring break, along with her "freshmates," as she called them, Ariel Massengale and Isabelle Harrison. "The froshies have been struggling with sleep lately because of so many tests and midterms. The teachers pile you up right before you leave for spring break. I'll be excited to sleep in."

Burdick also was eager to experience her first NCAA postseason. "I am excited to see what's ahead of us," she said. "I am excited to just get out on the floor and know it's one and done if we don't come out and produce. I am excited to see how far we go." The coaching staff was likely to stick with the all-senior starters. The decision should end the day-before-a-game exchanges between coaches and media, who wanted to list starters, that weren't intended to be evasive but were never specific. The truth was the coaches made game day decisions, sometimes based on health, and often because of practice performance and matchups. "In this program you still have to bring it in practice," Lockwood said. "If you have a toad practice, you're going to find yourself on a toadstool."

The seniors owned the outcome of the 2012 postseason. Regular starters Ariel Massengale, Taber Spani, Meighan Simmons, and on occasion, Burdick, had to adjust to roles off the bench. "Winning is a great cure-all," Lockwood said. "The buy-in in Nashville was great. One of things that excited us is we saw some maturing, some growing up in front of our eyes. There was some competitive maturity and one of the ways you define that is how people accept roles and moments like that. When people are happy for other people, even when things might not be perfect for themselves, that's a sign of maturity. I say this with more wishfulness than assurance, but hopefully that is taking place. We saw people being all-in for the team. It's all about what that scoreboard says when we walk off."

Massengale filled a position of high need as a point guard, so she logged what could be called starter minutes, even though she came off the bench. The coaches wanted to get Spani on the floor, but they also had to watch her closely. "Her issue is more mobility than performance," Lockwood said. "We watch how she is moving. We watch how she is running the floor. If she is not able to get acceleration, we tend to get her out quicker. If she is moving well, because she is such a smart player, and she is a kid who can knock down shots, we're more inclined when we see her move well to trust her more."

The coaches used the entire roster of 11 that season at various times, including all three freshmen. It could be a challenge for the coaches to spread out minutes and for players to accept roles. "One of the hardest things for coaches to communicate and for players to hear and embrace is (minutes played)," Lockwood said. "Rarely are 11 players going to get 15 minutes or more. It's just not going to happen. You tell players we need everybody to be ready, but at the same time we're going to make battlefield decisions. We'll see who's producing and that player or that group of players will get more minutes."

The senior lineup had hit its stride and so had the staff on the sideline. "As the season has gone on, our communication in that area has improved," Lockwood said "On the bench in the game it's rare you've got a whole lot of time. You've got seconds to make it." Warlick took more of the in-game coaching duties, and she was often on her feet shouting instructions to the team. Lockwood and DeMoss conferred about rotations and sought Summitt's input, and Summitt immediately endorsed some changes and said to wait on others. The coaches needed to find their rhythm, too, and substitutions had to remain flexible but also with the recognition that if a combination was working, it stayed on the court. "What we've emphasized to our team is that if there's any choice between a certain individual and the team's performance, that decision has been made a long time ago," Lockwood said. "We love them all, but it is about team performance."

One example was the Tennessee game against LSU in the SEC tourney title matchup. The five on the floor, with reserve Kamiko Williams playing a major role on the perimeter, seized control of the game. "At that point we weren't considering anyone else," Lockwood said. "That's going to happen. Those are game moments." That was where the coaches hoped the bench players bought in and realized their time was coming. It helped that the seniors were a close-knit group, with the underclassmen wanting to win for them. The underclassmen also knew those five would leave a huge void, and they had to get ready for the future.

"Being visual learners, which I think a lot of us are, and watching our seniors get out there and do their job and be the leaders on the floor, I think that's why we learned," Simmons said. "You visualize what your teammates are doing and don't make the same mistakes when you get out there. It's a learning experience rather than worrying about playing time, because next year we are going to be playing. We shouldn't have any worries, any doubts, nothing."

When Stricklen drained a three late against LSU to nearly seal the outcome in Nashville, Simmons danced along the sideline. "It just comes out," Simmons said. "The coaches expect us to be excited and into the game. But I think that kind of emotion—that is going to help us. We need to make sure we feed off of each other's energy." Lockwood would approve of the buying-in and the spontaneous sideline celebration. "It's our job," Lockwood said. "It's their game."

28

NCAA TOURNEY TIME

Media day at Allstate Arena featured the four sub-regional teams meeting with the press, with one coach saying Pat Summitt could come out of retirement to play again and another calling her the greatest in the game. After three years of coming up short when it came to the program's standard—the Final Four—the seniors intended to play with both focus and abandon. "Play every game like it's your last because it really is," Briana Bass said. Vicki Baugh earned a national title ring in 2008, but that postseason success seemed like a long time ago in 2012. "Any game can be your last. I want to play for Tennessee as long as possible," she said.

Meighan Simmons was headed into her second postseason and understood that the regular season didn't matter once the calendar flipped to March. "It is gone. The second time around I realize it's more about poise and patience, one game at a time." It was the last time around for Shekinna Stricklen, and she decided to release the anxiety and enjoy the process. Taber Spani also understood the weight of the expectations at Tennessee and how important it was to embrace them rather than be suffocated. The team gained a lot of confidence in Nashville during the SEC tourney and needed to tap into that source again. "We needed confidence," Spani said. "When our team plays confidently, we are tough to beat. We try not to focus on that (expectations) just because everyone else is, but we understand that we are playing for Pat and we are playing for this senior class."

What Tennessee hasn't done in the past three postseasons was a topic, but the staff wanted the players to change their approach. "The winner sees what he or she wants to do and accomplish," Lockwood said. "The loser focuses on what he or she wants to avoid. We don't want them thinking about what they want to avoid. We want them thinking about what they want to do." In 2012 Summitt used a postseason theme of catching a rabbit. If you scooted after several of the darting bunnies, you wouldn't catch a single one. But if you focused on one, you could scoop up that rabbit. That was the approach to each game. The first rabbit was Tennessee-Martin.

Coach Kevin McMillan, who was in his third season at UTM and had steered one of the youngest teams in college basketball to the NCAA tourney the previous season, had considerable success in 2012, too. The Skyhawks had won 14 consecutive games coming into Chicago. McMillan's concerns were the Lady Vols on the glass and Tennessee on the uniforms. "You saw the reaction when you asked the girls did they grow up watching Tennessee—well, there's no question," McMillan said. "We felt when we saw Tennessee come up that our biggest challenge would be taking that Tennessee name off that chest and just playing a basketball game."

The Skyhawks could drain three-pointers. Their weakness was on the boards, and that concerned the head coach. "They have got too many rebounders," McMillan said. "We've got one or two, three, but they've got five kids out there at any time that can kill you on the glass. If they're not executing well, or defending well, they are still going to kill you on the boards." Still, his players expressed nothing but excitement about playing the Lady Vols. "I love Tennessee; I've always watched Tennessee," said a beaming Heather Butler. "Since Candace Parker, and even further beyond that, I've watched them ever since I was in middle school. I've always wanted to play against Tennessee and am very glad that we get this opportunity to go out on the floor with them."

McMillan put together a tough non-conference schedule for his team—the slate included NCAA participants Purdue, Louisville, and Vanderbilt—and the Skyhawks were able to compete against teams with more talent because they could shoot the ball. "They shoot a lot of threes," Holly Warlick said. "We have not been known to defend the three ball very well, so it's

going to be a huge challenge for us. We are not taking this game lightly."
Tennessee-Martin averaged 27 three-point attempts per game. "They'll
shoot them in quick transition," Dean Lockwood said. "They'll drive and
kick. They set a ton of ball screens. They are awful good. When they can spot
up four players who can all shoot the ball with a great deal of effectiveness,
it's hard. Defenses are so trained to help. If there is dribble penetration or
someone is attacking, even one step (by the defender) and a kick, you're
curtains."

The team's commitment to the long ball reminded Lockwood of Rick
Pitino bursting on the scene with Providence—and getting the Friars to a
Final Four in 1987—by calculating that three points, if a team makes enough
of them, will outpace twos over the course of a game.

"They live and die," Lockwood said. "They are going to try and beat you
with threes."

Tennessee needed long-ball scoring from Stricklen, preferably to start
the game, rather than arriving in the second half. Alicia Manning said the
players did some introspective work with a psychological bent, and the
team's recent analysis revealed the need to be intense as opposed to tense.
It was a message Stricklen needed, and to some extent, Manning needed it,
too. "Tense means you're apprehensive and fearful about your performance
a little bit," Lockwood said. "You worry about outcomes. (Stricklen) said,
'Sometimes when I miss my first couple of shots, I get a little (hesitant).'
I said, 'You can get tense about it, which is not productive at all, or stay
intense, where you are in the moment, you are very focused, you believe in
yourself, and you know great shooters have that mentality that the next ball
is going in.'"

Lockwood compared it to traversing unfamiliar territory. There are reasons to be cautious, but don't lose confidence. "It's almost like walking up a
blind, dark alley," Lockwood said. "Intense is, 'I'm very focused, but I'm very
confident. If something happens I have a plan. Or if that plan fails I have a
Plan B.' So, I am intense, I am very tuned in, but I am not at all worried or
fearful." When Stricklen hit a deep three-pointer against South Carolina
in the quarterfinals of the SEC tourney, she let loose a scream as she ran
down the court. "Showing that exuberance, she was like a kid and someone
just fed her a packet of Kool-Aid," Lockwood said. "We want that, and we
don't want her to be fearful of outcomes. We want her to trust herself and
say, 'I am a good player. I am going to make this play. No fear.'"

Getting Manning to loosen up paid dividends, too. She had always been
a steady rebounder and hustle player, but Manning scored in the SEC

tourney, hitting a trey in each of the three games, and kept the defenses honest. Lockwood noted that at times Manning's arms could get so rigid as to resemble steel cables. "At times she tries too hard. You can self-sabotage. It's like the baseball pitcher who says, 'Don't throw it high and wide. Don't throw it high and wide. Don't throw it high and wide.' Sure enough, when you think about what you want to avoid and not do, you end up almost flipping the script on yourself. Relax, take a deep breath, look around, enjoy this, and go play."

Tennessee-Martin was likely better than a 15 seed—earlier bracket projections had them as a 13—but the committee may have found matching the Lady Vols with Pat Summitt's alma mater too tempting. On the third page of the Skyhawks' game notes was a photo of Summitt scoring for UTM, which was known then as the Lady Pacers. The photo noted that Summitt, who played from 1970 to 1974, held the single-game record of 35 points—a record that was broken that season by Heather Butler, who poured in 42 against Tennessee State, and got to 1,000 career points in 50 games, whereas Summitt did so in 59.

The Lady Vols tipped the game in Chicago on March 17, St. Patrick's Day. The second game featured DePaul and BYU. Chicago is DePaul's hometown, but the Blue Demons play on campus near downtown, while Allstate is in Rosemont. "Daggumit, we've got to go up against St. Patrick's Day in Chicago," DePaul Coach Doug Bruno said. "We all love St. Patrick's Day in Chicago."

It was unseasonably warm in the Windy City with temperatures in the 70s that weekend. That time of year usually brings cold weather, even snow in Chicago. Vicki Baugh, whose surgically repaired knee feels better when it's warm, welcomed the climate. "I am praising the weather gods right now," Baugh said.

No player was happier to be in Chicago than Ariel Massengale, who is from nearby Bolingbrook. Each player gets an allotment of postseason tickets for family and friends, but Massengale's need exceeded supply, so she sent a text asking teammates for any unused ones. Several players offered to help, including fellow freshmen Cierra Burdick and Isabelle Harrison, and she was able to compile a ticket list of 20. "I gave her all my tickets almost," Harrison said. "This is her hometown." Burdick had been giving her friend a hard time about Tennessee getting Chicago—a native of North Carolina, she had hoped for Chapel Hill in the sub-regional—but she made a ticket donation. "Don't hurt my heart," Burdick said when reminded that Tennessee went north instead of east. Burdick had become a go-to player for quotes. She took a swig of orange juice right before the interview started and then made a nasty face. She had just brushed her teeth. "Toothpaste and orange juice, ugh," Burdick said.

Burdick had driven Massengale to Summitt's house for the Selection Show when Massengale had shrieked with joy over the Chicago site. "I was contemplating making her walk home, but I've forgiven her," Burdick said. Massengale had dozens of supporters in the stands, from high school friends to other family members and fans who bought their own ducats. Several other Lady Vols had familiar faces in the seats, too. Briana Bass' family made the trip from relatively nearby Indianapolis. Shekinna Stricklen had relatives traveling from Arkansas, and Meighan Simmons also had two friendly faces in the stands—her Steele High School coach and the coach's husband, who made the trip from Cibolo, Texas.

Vicki Baugh had family in Chicago–when she drove to Knoxville from Sacramento in August of 2007 to begin her college career, the Windy City was a stopover to rest and visit before continuing to Tennessee. Those family members would be in attendance.

"My grandfather's family is from here," said Baugh, who wanted to have her car while in college, so she made the cross-country trek to get it to the Volunteer State.

The media have access to the locker rooms during the NCAA tourney, and the reporters typically interview the players directly before practice. Taber Spani could not sit still, even in the locker room during the open media portion. The team was scheduled to practice as soon as their press duties were done that Friday before the game, and Spani sat in front of her locker, her right foot tapping the floor like a metronome. "It's just me wanting to get ready," Spani said. "I just do it. I don't know why."

It was an interesting locker room with modern wall décor, wood accents, and blue metal lockers that looked circa 1950. The press conference area was held in an annex building that is across the street from the arena, but nobody had to go outside: a long tunnel that goes under the street connects the arena and the building, and a golf cart ferried the coaches and players back and forth. When the golf cart slowed uphill, the hyperkinetic Glory Johnson jumped off and pushed it from behind.

Spani had that same energy, and her right leg never stopped moving in the locker room. Her left leg still had a brace on the knee. "The first two years going in and then having it taken away (by losses in the Sweet 16 and Elite Eight), I learned how much it really does matter," Spani said. "You have two great regular seasons, great start to postseason, and then it ends.

We're at a program where the NCAA and what you do and the results of that define a legacy and how a team comes together. This is everything."

The support for Summitt poured in that day from the other three coaches in the sub-regional. McMillan had the quip of the day when he was asked how the Skyhawks would try to handle the Lady Vols on the glass. "We're going to see if they will allow us to play with six, and we've told Coach Summitt we have her jersey in our locker room if she wants to put it on and help us, as the last time Tennessee-Martin beat Tennessee, she was playing," McMillan said. BYU Coach Jeff Judkins spoke to Summitt at the arena. "She is a legend. I think that every coach respects what she has done and the way that she runs her program. As a coach she loves the game. Another part I like is that she's got some fire. I really like that. She's not afraid to say how she feels to her team."

Bruno has known Summitt for years and issued an unequivocal endorsement. "This is the greatest coach in the history of our sport. Not just the greatest women's coach. This is 1,000 wins. She doesn't get recognized without it being qualified—she's won a thousand women's games. She's won a thousand college games. She is the winningest coach in the sport of college basketball. She's been so much more than just Tennessee's great coach."

29

SUCCESS IN CHICAGO

Meighan Simmons sat on the back of a golf cart and hollered for Glory Johnson to hurry up. The motorized vehicle, which ferried the players and coaches down and up a ramp to connect Allstate Arena to the Skyline Room, already had Simmons and Holly Warlick on board. Johnson bolted out of the locker room and was whisked away to the press conference.

It was one of the few times that Johnson needed to get in gear in Tennessee's 72–49 win over UTM, the alma mater of Pat Summitt, in a game attended by 4,161 on St. Patrick's Day in the Windy City. The senior tallied a double-double with 14 points and 12 rebounds. "We face double teams, we face teams sagging off us, but Glory is our go-to player and we rely on her to make plays and she has the ability to go up and get the ball with two, three people on her," Warlick said. "We want Glory to make plays and we want her involved in the offense. Any great post player, if they don't touch the ball a few times down the floor, then post players may tend to quit working, but Glory keeps working. She is the exception to that rule."

Simmons did her part, too. "We tried to get the ball inside, but if you watch they were not defending our point guard, they were not extending their defense, they were really packing it in, so it was really difficult to get the ball inside. And credit to them—they were physical, they played very tough, so we had to hit shots to open up the inside," Warlick said. "Credit to Meighan, she hit some big shots, some big threes, which really opened up the inside for us." The sophomore led all scorers with 20 points and was 4–7 from long range. "You know Meighan is an awesome shooter," said Kamiko Williams, who entered the game eight minutes into the first half because she can put the ball on the floor and get to the paint, which the Lady Vols needed when shots didn't fall to start the game. Tennessee needed the offensive boost, as the Lady Vols struggled to connect to start the game. The Lady Vols attempted 16 three-pointers in the first half and made just four of them—one each from Stricklen, Manning, Massengale, and Simmons.

UTM didn't have much success either. The Skyhawks rely on the long ball, and they were 3–12 from long range before the break. The Lady Vols played an aggressive man and switching defense and used their length to disrupt UTM. Their leading scorers, Heather Butler and Jasmine Newsome—who averaged 44 points per game combined—tallied 24 total, and were a combined 8–43 from the field overall and 1–13 from the arc. "Tennessee is kind of a cumulative effect," UTM Coach Kevin McMillan said. "It is a wear down, wear down, wear down, so it's hard to make those shots as you get worn down. That is what they do that is going to cause those problems, and if you add in that you just missed a few open shots, then you have a snowball. But their defense is relentless and pounding on you."

UTM led 7–5 at the 16:39 mark of the first half when Jaclissa Haislip connected on a three-pointer. Stricklen put Tennessee ahead, 8–7, on a three-pointer at the 14:10 mark, and the Lady Vols never trailed again. Tennessee built the lead to 17–9 when Williams drove and dished to Stricklen and then 19–11 when Williams drove and connected on an elbow jumper. Williams was deployed for defense in the last game of the SEC tourney, and she was inserted for offense in the first game of the NCAA tourney. With UTM packing the paint, the Lady Vols needed a guard who could disrupt that setup inside, and Williams delivered with three assists in 12 minutes of play in the first half. "Holly was like, 'Miko, penetrate, get to the paint,'" Williams said. "I was like, 'OK, Coach, I got you.' That is my game. We had to get to the basket. They were doubling down on Vicki and Glory."

Johnson's nickname could be "Christmas Tree" because the forward spent most of the game trying to score with players, ornaments as it were,

hanging on her. Johnson and Baugh, who gets uptight when smaller players hover around her surgically repaired knee, were visibly frustrated, and
Williams helped Johnson by delivering a pep talk. "I tell her, 'You've got it.
You're the best post, I think personally, in the nation. So, just go out there
and do your thing. Can't nobody stop you.'" Williams played with Johnson
in AAU basketball when both were in high school, and she was impressed
with how Johnson held her cool on the court despite all the body blows she
absorbed. "She has gotten a whole lot better," Williams said. "I remember in
AAU she used to just blow up. Now, she just walks out of there. She knows
we need her, so she keeps her composure."

The smaller team did what it had to do–sagged into the paint and left
jump shooters open on the perimeter. Tennessee showed patience at first;
after at least six passes, Alicia Manning connected on a trey ball and a 3–0
start for the Lady Vols. But then the Lady Vols were tempted by how open
they were, and shots were lofted from all over the court by every player on
the floor. Had the shots fallen, the game would have been over in the first
10 minutes, but the Lady Vols weren't connecting. An assortment of players checked in and they all found the openness appealing. And nearly all of
them misfired.

Pat Summitt had seen enough late in the first half and called timeout.
But she didn't unload on the players. Instead, they were told to be patient
and get better shots. "Pat Summitt has not quit coaching, and so she is just
more focused on one-on-one, individual help, so I am sure she was trying
to get a couple kids' attention," Warlick said. "You don't have to worry about
Pat not coaching and getting the point across, whether it is praise or giving
them a swift kick in the butt."

Briana Bass misfired on a long ball a few minutes into the second half,
but Manning got the rebound and got the ball to Baugh, who fired it right
back to Bass with orders to shoot. Bass swished that one. "Strick told me she
was going to beat me up if I kept hesitating, so I've got to do something,"
Bass said. "I really was," Shekinna Stricklen confirmed. "Teams are going
to leave her open until she can prove that she can score. She is one of the
best shooters, and she's got to have the confidence to just let it go."

UTM's intent was to foul inside and send the Lady Vols to the line, but the
officials didn't make the calls. "They funny thing is that one of our strategies
was that we were going to foul their players in the paint," McMillan said.
"We only committed 12. And we were trying to foul." McMillan wanted to
send Tennessee to the line as opposed to a track meet where the Lady Vols
would use their speed in the open floor and their size to get to the rim. But

the whistles rarely blew on either end, and once the Lady Vols settled down, they built a comfortable lead, took the win, and got to the second round to play DePaul, on March 19, 2012. DePaul dispatched BYU to get to the second round.

The last time Tennessee played DePaul, Williams and Ariel Massengale sat beside each other on the bench and watched. Neither could check into the December 11, 2011, game in Madison Square Garden due to injury. Bruno was aware of their absence, and he noted that Tennessee's game in December seemed to be one of experimentation at point guard with Stricklen playing the bulk of her minutes at the spot. He also knew the availability of the pair made the Lady Vols a better team in March. "I think they used our game in December to see what Stricklen could do up top if that was the way it was going to have to go," Bruno said. DePaul had dealt with its own injury issues and, after the loss of All-American Keisha Hampton in January 2012, was left with seven players to finish the season. The Blue Demons regrouped, stayed competitive in the Big East, and earned a berth in the NCAA tourney.

Players and coaches from both teams said the game in December was rather meaningless in March. "We're just trying to survive and advance," DePaul senior guard Deanna Ortiz said. "We're a different team than we were in December; they're a different team." Massengale chatted with Chanise Jenkins, a freshman point guard for DePaul who also didn't play in the December game because of injury. Jenkins, who is from Chicago, ended up taking a redshirt year. "I wish that she was playing, because it would be really neat for us to play against each other and to be playing in Chicago," Massengale said.

Taber Spani noted that the team would look familiar on film because the style of play remained the same, offering some benefit to a rematch. "It matters in the sense that we have an idea of what they run, and we can go back and look at that tape, and look at what we did well and what we need to improve on, so that matters," Spani said. "But we're a completely different team now and two months down the road everybody looks different, and obviously we have a lot more to play for, too. That can't really be measured by a game in the past."

Some of the best parts for the media about being in a sub-regional with Bruno were the entertaining press conferences. He joked that Michael Fahey, the video coordinator for Tennessee, didn't even have a job after graduating from Benedictine in 2010 and somehow got to work for the Lady Vols. Fahey, who is close friends with the Bruno family, worked for the Indiana Fever as a video specialist before taking the job with Tennessee for the 2011–12 season. Bruno also gave his synopsis of "The Magnificent Seven," which he used to describe his seven remaining players, though he noted they didn't always play that magnificently. Any media members who knew the movie in the press conference dated themselves—the western film was released in 1960—and the DePaul band had started playing the theme song. Bruno also noted that the father of guard Anna Martin, who is from Nicholasville, Kentucky, suggested a treatment of Epsom salt and moonshine for the injured players. Bruno said he approved the salts but not the 'shine.

The coach was a member of the Glory Johnson Fan Club and said too much was made with regard to timing when it came to board play. He said Johnson rebounded the best way—with her eyes. "She's probably the most relentless rebounder in the country," Bruno said. "She just really, really pursues the glass with a vigor that is kind of in remembrance of what all the Tennessee players in the program have been about. They've always been great rebounders, and Glory is really, really active and really, really tough to keep off the glass." Johnson made Bruno look like a prophet. She grabbed a career high of 21 rebounds, and the Lady Vols stiffened their defense with a 63–48 win over DePaul in a physical battle at Allstate Arena. The nearly 3,000 fans in attendance seemed bewildered at the lack of whistles, stating their objections loudly, but the players pushed through it on both sides. "That's something you have to get used to," Johnson said. "It's a big girl's game."

The Lady Vols earned a trip to the Des Moines Regional in Iowa, where they would meet Kansas in the Sweet 16. Baylor and Georgia Tech joined them in that regional, with the winner headed to Denver for the Final Four. It was well past midnight Eastern Time when the Lady Vols finished the post-game press conference in Chicago, and they took a charter plane back to Knoxville as soon as they finished. Tips times in the NCAA tourney are set by TV contracts, not the benefit of student-athletes or media with deadlines. The losing team went first, so Bruno addressed the media while Warlick sat in a holding room, off limits to even the Knoxville media. All three Knoxville television stations were in Chicago, as were the beat writers for *InsideTennessee* and the *Knoxville News Sentinel*, but the NCAA official on-site rebuffed their pleas to interview Warlick. The media could see her, and she was willing to talk if allowed, but they could not approach her. It was a maddening situation.

Postseason always meant teams had to grind out games, and the Lady Vols were up to the challenge in Chicago. "We haven't played a real pretty game in a while," Mickie DeMoss said. "This is not a real pretty-type team in that we win pretty. But it's a win. It's a grind. And we made stops when we had to make stops and made baskets when we had to make baskets." Tennessee led 28–23 at halftime with an offensive boost off the bench from Simmons, who tallied 12 points before the break. Johnson was controlling the boards for Tennessee but having trouble scoring. Baugh stepped in to fill that void for the Lady Vols. "With Glory not scoring, the fact that Vicki could step up and provide that scoring for us inside was huge," DeMoss said.

Baugh scored the last basket of the game with a layup assisted by Spani, and Johnson grabbed the ball after a missed basket by DePaul with 11 seconds left—an appropriate way to end the game. It was Johnson's 21st rebound of the game. Her previous career high had been 18 against Mississippi State in January with her NCAA high at 14 against Notre Dame in March of 2011. Each one had been hard earned. From Johnson's point of view, she wasn't scoring, so she needed to contribute in another way. Simmons sat in her locker and was speechless for a moment as she stared at Johnson's stat line of 21 rebounds. "I have nothing to say," Simmons said, looking at the interviewer and back down at the box score as if to reconfirm the number. "That's an OK night," Dean Lockwood deadpanned.

"She was getting hammered every single time she tried to do a putback, but she stayed with it, she stayed composed and made sure that she didn't let it get to her, and she just continued to play," Simmons said.

That composure had been a work in progress for Johnson, and she fully arrived during her senior season. Johnson struggled as a freshman with how much contact was allowed in college. "My whole attitude and demeanor has developed over time and that is something I can thank my teammates for and my coaches," Johnson said. "They keep me composed. As a freshman, that wasn't going to happen. All I knew was that if someone hit me, I was going to hit them back."

Massengale's parents were easy to find at the arena with their No. 5 T-shirts. Her boisterous aunt, who wore a "We Back Pat" T-shirt, was easy to hear as she was on her feet cheering and letting her niece know about it after a turnover. "She is like that all the time," Massengale said. "Growing up she came to all my state tournaments in high school. She is like my daddy. They put their critiques in after a game."

The Lady Vols did not take any style points home from Chicago, but they did head back to Knoxville with two wins and a trip to the Sweet 16 on the travel itinerary. The Lady Vols had to grind out the victories at Allstate Arena, and they prevailed by playing the Tennessee Way—with strong defense and rebounding. Postseason whistles tend to go silent, but in the Chicago subregional the officials almost could have called the game without any whistles at all. The contact was constant, and Johnson made her way to the rim with Blue Demons draped on her and holding her jersey. While she made few shots, she got on the boards. "It's going to be a long flight home," a weary and sore Johnson said after the game.

"Glory is an incredible player with incredible athletic ability," Baugh said. "I said it earlier that there's nothing she can't do and I wasn't worried that she wasn't scoring points because she's always going to bring an all-around game—defense, rebounding, pushing the ball, running in transition. She does it all. She's going to find a way to play strong and get through it and make it work one way or another." Baugh picked up the slack on the scoreboard with an 8–11 performance from the field and 17 points. Her buckets came from getting to the rim and finishing, and she got the lead to double digits early in the second half when she saw DePaul's post player, Katherine Harry, chasing shooters on the perimeter. Baugh slipped to the top of the paint, called for the ball, got it before Harry could recover, and went right to the basket. She got a steal in the open floor two minutes later and headed all the way to the rim for a 39–27 lead. Meanwhile, Stricklen had four assists by finding players in transition, including Baugh late in the second half. Stricklen also found Briana Bass early in the second half for a three-pointer.

But it was Tennessee's defense that was the difference in Chicago. The Lady Vols faced two teams that liked the three ball: UTM led the nation in scoring and launched 27 treys a game, while DePaul made nearly eight three-pointers a game and entered the game against the Lady Vols three shy of the program's single season record. UTM was 4–20 (20.0 percent) while DePaul was 3–17 (17.6 percent). The Blue Demons got the school record of 256 treys in a single season, besting the 2010–11 team with 255, but they tallied five under their average for a game. Brittany Hrynko and Megan Rogowski, who had combined for 101 three-pointers in the 2011–12 season, were a combined 0–11 from long range against Tennessee. Neither team Tennessee faced in Chicago reached 50 points. UTM was averaging 81.1 points, while DePaul scored 72.8 points per game.

"It starts with the seniors," Johnson said. "It's our responsibility and that's one thing that we take pride in—our defense and our rebounding—because that's what the program is based off of and that's what we've learned since we were freshmen coming in."

30

POSTS READY FOR POSTSEASON

The Lady Vols got back on the practice court in Knoxville, and Glory Johnson bore the marks of a hard-fought sub-regional in Chicago. Johnson was her usual energetic self, but she had visible scratches and bruises on her arms and shoulders after two physical showdowns inside Allstate Arena. "She stepped up big for us," Pat Summitt said.

The team's plane didn't arrive back in Knoxville until nearly 3 a.m. Tuesday, so the coaches gave the players a rest day and then got back inside Pratt Pavilion on Wednesday. "Physical and late-night arrival, so both of those things," Dean Lockwood said by way of explanation. By waiting until Wednesday, the coaches also knew who the next opponent would be since Kansas didn't play until Tuesday evening. "You can always work on yourself, but it does help when you can focus a little bit more, and you can tell them some specifics, especially this time of year," Lockwood said. It was also the time of year when Lockwood loses his voice, which was raspy and at considerably lower volume. "After 30 years of coaching the vocal cords have gotten weak," Lockwood said. "This is all I've got."

Pat Summitt wasn't too pleased with the team's practice session Wednesday. "Just a little disappointing today. At this time of the year, you worry about everything, as coaches. I don't think they were worried about anything," Summitt said with a smile. "They will come back and be better. Coach DeMoss kind of chewed on them a little bit." The Lady Vols practiced again Thursday and then departed for Iowa, where they were joined by Kansas, Georgia Tech, and Baylor. Kansas earned the trip by taking out Delaware on Tuesday. Baylor eliminated Florida, while Georgia Tech dispatched Georgetown. There had been some criticism in some quarters about whether or not Kansas deserved a bid to the Big Dance, but the Jayhawks answered it with wins over Nebraska and Delaware. A team that feels disrespected—and responds—could be a very dangerous one.

"Can anyone say VCU men's basketball?" Lockwood noted. "Once you are in it, you are in it. It doesn't matter how you got there. We knew they were on the bubble with 19 wins. I think they have more than proved that they belong in this tournament."

In 2011, VCU became the first team to advance from the "First Four" to the Final Four. The men's NCAA tourney had expanded that year to 68 teams with four selected for "play-in" games. VCU, an 11 seed, took out No. 1 seed Kansas to win the Southwest Region in San Antonio, Texas, and advance to the Final Four in Houston. VCU would fall to Butler, a No. 8 seed and fellow improbable participant in the Final Four, in the semifinal.

Taber Spani, who is from the Midwest—her hometown is Lee's Summit, Missouri—was beaming when talking about Iowa. It would be a relatively short drive for her family in the Kansas City area to head north about 200 miles to get to Des Moines. "I can't wait to get on that plane and go," Spani said. "I am so excited."

Tipoff was set for 11:04 a.m. local time, so the Lady Vols would be up early for the game as opposed to waiting all day, like they did in Chicago for Monday's game against DePaul that started at 9:40 p.m. Eastern Time. "We have played at all times so we know how to prepare regardless of if it's early or late," Vicki Baugh said. "As long as the weather is good I think we will be fine." This was Baugh's first trip to the Hawkeye State. "I don't know what to expect," she said. "I have a friend that went to school there and that is about the only thing I can associate with Iowa." The weather forecast was in Baugh's favor—the warmer the weather, the better her knee felt. It was spring-like weather in Des Moines, which is very unusual for late March, with trees blooming around the downtown Wells Fargo Arena and temperatures in the 70s during the day.

Doug Bruno was very aware of Baugh's surgical history, and while he may have been on the opponent's bench, he had nothing but respect for the Tennessee forward. He was the head coach for the 2006 USA U18 FIBA Americas and the 2007 FIBA U19 World Championship Team, both of which won gold medals (the 2006 squad went 4–0 in Colorado; the 2007 USA team went 9–0 in Slovakia). Baugh, who was still in high school, played on those teams and left a lasting impression on Bruno. "She broke the rim dunking after practice one day," Bruno said. Baugh became one of Bruno's favorite players. He was effusive in his praise of the Sacramento native and said she would have been an All-American in college had it not been for the two ACL surgeries on her left knee.

When she played USA ball in 2006, Baugh was one of three high school players on a team of college players. The other two high schoolers were Maya Moore and Kayla Pedersen. Bruno said some of the experienced players were not as easy to reach—he indicated that they acted as if they had the answers already—and it was "very impressive to see Maya, Vicki, and Kayla stand up and say, 'This is how we do things.' The maturity of these players, especially Vicki. . . . When you're the youngest, it's easy to get swept along," Bruno said.

"I remember we were willing to work, specifically those three players," Baugh said of the high school trio. "We just wanted to learn. We knew it was a new experience because it was for us, and I remember being very open to everything he had to say and wanting to learn. There were older cats there—that is who he is talking about—and they had experience already. I think we ended up starting over them, and it was kind of weird because nobody expected it."

Baugh's career at Tennessee was truncated by injuries, but some of her best moments came in postseason, starting in Tampa in 2008 when her drive to the basket (the one that tore the ACL in her left knee for the first time) gave the Lady Vols a double-digit lead in the national title game against Stanford. As Baugh was being helped from the court, she had tears streaming down her face and she yelled at the Tennessee bench, "Let's go, y'all!" It was a moment that galvanized the team, which maintained the lead and trimmed the nets for the program's eighth national title.

Baugh's words entered Lady Vol lore, and a lasting image of Nicky Anosike was seeing her wipe tears from her eyes when she re-took the court in Tampa. Anosike, who wore No. 55 at Tennessee, switched her jersey in the WNBA to No. 21 in a salute to Baugh. "She has got a great heart and a great heart for people," said Lockwood, who was one of those who helped to get Baugh off the court in 2008. "She is very quiet by nature and for a lot of people it probably takes time to get a feel or a sense of who Vicki is as a person, to get the essence of her. She is very, very caring. She has got a depth to her and a quality to her that is very, very special."

Baugh was effective in the sub-regional in Chicago in the wins over Tennessee-Martin and DePaul. In the 63–48 win over DePaul that got the Lady Vols to Des Moines, Glory Johnson was all over the glass with 21 rebounds but was having trouble scoring. Baugh filled the offensive void and went 8–11 for 16 points and also had nine rebounds. "I am playing and I am not thinking too much and that is the good thing about it," Baugh said. "I thought I had missed a bunch that game. I didn't realize I was 8–11. I told myself that I am going to keep shooting and every shot I take are shots that I think I can make."

Lockwood smiled after that game when asked if it was a good time to be the post coach between Baugh's work on the scoreboard and Johnson's performance on the glass. He also hoped that Baugh's offense was packed for Iowa. "Vicki defensively is certainly a game changer for us. But when Vicki's offense is going—and that is one of the things we challenged her with at halftime—when she is converting like she did in the second half, our team goes up a full notch. She is athletic and she has got the skill set to score. When she brings that, it is like adding another ship to your fleet."

It was her USA Basketball play that introduced Baugh to Bruno, and the respect was mutual. "USA was very tough, and I remember a few of the girls even breaking down because he is very strict and stern, and it is business on the court. I even remember we had to rehearse—and it was kind of like a military thing—and he called them 'We Wills,' that were basically 10 commitments that we will do before every game and every practice," Baugh said. "I remember having three-a-days. I think some of us who were stronger surprised him because we were able to handle it."

There was a moment in the DePaul game when Baugh's momentum carried her out of bounds toward the Blue Demons bench. She got her balance and needed to turn down court, and Bruno stepped forward onto the court to give her additional room. Baugh darted behind Bruno and headed to the other end. "I know he did that to make sure that I was OK. I even saw their bench step back. I tripped over someone (on the court), and I was falling out of bounds, stumbling, and trying to recover. He is a very caring guy. He still checks on me to this day."

31

MEDIA DAY IN DES MOINES

The day before regional play begins in the NCAA Tournament, the teams meet with the media, who conduct interviews and watch a portion of the beginning of practice. With Pat Summitt on the court, the baseline was lined with photographers.

The Lady Vol locker room was crowded that Friday, March 23, during the open time for the press with representatives from national media, including *The New York Times*; a contingent from Knoxville, including the television stations; and the local Iowa press. The media even included the AARP, and its representatives—one had a boom mic—pitched questions to players and coaches about Summitt and her decision to coach this season after announcing that she had early onset dementia. The question about Summitt's future had been a popular one with the media. Dean Lockwood was asked what his call would be if he were a betting man, He offered a passionate endorsement of Summitt that went well beyond her ability to coach.

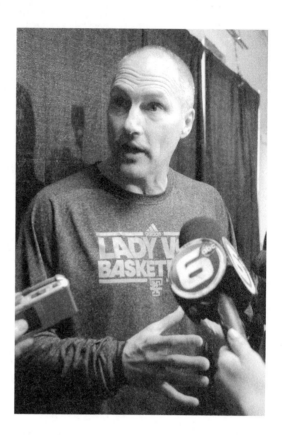

Assistant Coach Dean Lockwood handled additional media duties during the final season and became a go-to for the sports press.

"I am not a betting man, so I am a terrible guy to ask that question," Lockwood said. "I would just tell you that Coach has so much passion for this game. I have not been around a lot more competitive people, if any, than Pat Summitt. One of the things that she is more passionate about than anything is mentoring young women. I have no idea what her plan is on the immediate horizon, but I would tell you I would be very, very surprised if she wasn't involved in this program as a leader, as a mentor in some capacity doing something for Tennessee Lady Vol basketball.

"She is an incredible person of character. As great of a coach as she is, she is a caring woman. One of the hard things about coaching is to be tough on people and to be demanding on people. I give Pat so much credit because I am sure she knows there are times when players are irritated, aggravated, probably go home and say, 'That crazy woman.' But you know what? She has just taken a stand to mentor young women and to help young women be leaders and to be prepared for a lifetime of challenges whatever may lie ahead. In 38 years she has not wavered. And I have so much respect for that. I can't tell you how much I respect a person who is not concerned about what people think but about doing it the right way."

Kansas Coach Bonnie Henrickson first crossed paths with Summitt in Knoxville while working a summer camp for Tennessee. Henrickson was a graduate assistant at Western Illinois and had played Division II basketball at St. Cloud State, so she wasn't expecting interaction with Summitt at a camp attended by hundreds who were all vying for the coach's attention. "She took a moment to visit with me and speak to me, and she didn't have to do it," Henrickson said. "I have admired and respected how she has handled success. I have never gotten the sense from Pat that success defines who she is. Pat is an unbelievably loving, giving, compassionate person. To me, that is the most impressive thing."

Since Baylor was in Des Moines, another figure loomed large in the regional—the 6'8" Brittney Griner. The junior was a dominant force in college basketball that season, and some speculation had started that she would forego her senior year. Baylor Coach Kim Mulkey rather emphatically declared that Griner would return. Candace Parker was subject to endless speculation about her status in 2007 that continued even after she said she would return, and Mulkey sounded as if she were weary with the topic. She noted Griner wanted to leave with a college degree.

Henrickson, whose team was an 11 seed, was asked why it was not as common in the women's tourney for lower-seeded teams to get deep in the tourney as it was on the men's side. She noted that male players exiting for the NBA could equalize talent to some degree for the lower-seeded teams from smaller conferences. "It is more about the guys leaving early, the one and done, two and done," Henrickson said. "Then, you have some mid-major seniors who can make a freshman look silly at this time of the year. That kind of experience, or not having that, is a difference." The reporter cited teams such as Butler and VCU making the Final Four in 2011. "Ouch, don't say VCU to Kansas," Henrickson said with a smile, referring to VCU eliminating the Jayhawks in 2011 on the men's side in the Elite Eight. Henrickson also noted that situation is not the case for the women's game, but that Griner was welcome to make the leap. Kansas plays in the Big 12 and has to face Baylor in league play. "Don't tell Kim I said that," Henrickson joked.

Taber Spani felt right at home in the Midwest. The native of the Kansas City area had been smiling since Tennessee advanced to the Des Moines Regional. Spani smiled when asked if her offense was packed for the trip.

"It's coming back," Spani said. "I think sometimes for me I want it to go in too bad. I just sort of will my shot in instead of just not thinking and shooting." All Spani had to do to get a scouting report was call her older sister, Shalin Spani, who played for Kansas State. "I talked to her. They know Kansas very well. K-State beat them earlier." Spani's parents and younger sisters were still involved in high school basketball, so Tennessee had to get a Sweet 16 win for the Spanis to make the relatively short trip to Iowa for an Elite Eight game. That was extra motivation for Spani, because a win over Kansas meant a visit with family.

Spani was on the floor to stretch the defense because she can hit long-range threes. Spani also had the size to box out—she may not be able to grab the rebound, but she would make sure to check out an opponent, who wouldn't get it either. That meant the post players could box out another post and have a clearer path to the board rather than also have to fight off an incoming guard that didn't get picked up on the perimeter.

Glory Johnson, who had those career-high 21 rebounds, had the Jayhawks' attention. "We're going to do drills in practice to be able to stay focused, box out, and not try to just go for the ball, but be able to see her before we (go after) the ball," Kansas forward Aishah Sutherland said. Kansas had regrouped after losing leading scorer Carolyn Davis in mid-February to a torn ACL and dislocated left knee. "The initial reaction is how gut-wrenching it is for those players," Henrickson said. "Your heart goes out to Carolyn, obviously, and you turn around and circle the players, because they all know what that meant. . . . You can't let what you don't have keep you from using what you do have."

The loss of the junior forward's 16.9 points per game could have doomed Kansas, but the Jayhawks got even more from point guard Angel Goodrich. Henrickson first saw Goodrich play as an eighth-grader. "I thought she could help us then," Henrickson said, before adding with a smile, "but I couldn't convince her high school or parents to move her to Lawrence." Goodrich, who led the nation in assists with 244 and a career total of 520, logged a lot of minutes in 2012. Her stat line in minutes since the Big 12 season started on January 4 was: 40, 40, 47, 38, 40, 39, 39, 34, 44, 39, 37, 40, 39, 40, 39, 34, 40, 40, 40, 39, 40.

"Yeah, that is a lot of time," Goodrich said. "When I get to the media (timeout), I try to control my breathing, try to get my breath back. It's just whatever it takes to help my teammates get a win." Henrickson rarely pulled Goodrich in games, but she did in practice repetitions. If Goodrich made a mistake during her shift, she policed herself. "If she misses a layup or misses a box out and turns it over in practice, when she's subbed out, she runs down and back," Henrickson said. "I never say a word to her, and that makes everyone else do that as well."

Kansas got an at-large bid to the NCAA tourney and took out No. 6 seed Nebraska and No. 3 seed Delaware in order to reach Des Moines. "It all goes back to when Carolyn went down and we went through the emotion of all that—to circle the wagons and know that the goals and expectations weren't going to change," Henrickson said. "Life isn't about the hand that you have been dealt but the way you play the hand." Tennessee had changed its hand, and it started on Senior Day when the Lady Vols opened with the five seniors and stuck with the lineup in postseason. Tennessee was now 6–0 with the seniors, and freshman Cierra Burdick noted that it was them she was playing for. "I want to see them get to a Final Four," Burdick said. "I want to see them put all the negative criticism to rest. This is their last year and it's a great year for it to be done. It is a great deal of motivation. I love my seniors."

With Tennessee on spring break, the three freshmen had to move out of their dormitory and stay in a downtown Knoxville hotel. That meant Burdick, Ariel Massengale, and Isabelle Harrison had been in hotels in Chicago, Knoxville, and now Des Moines since March 16. "We can go to our teammates' house, but I still want my own room like I have at the dorm," Harrison said. "I have all my stuff packed." Still, it wasn't as bad as when the current seniors were freshmen. Summitt had booted them from the locker room after a desultory loss in February 2009, and they also lost laundry service—the managers get all the practice clothes ready each day—so they had to tote their gear back and forth and wash practice shorts and shirts in the hotel bathroom during spring break. The freshmen heard all about it from the seniors. "That was a rough time," Harrison said. "They tell us a lot of stories from their freshman year. A lot of stories. And I don't ever want those past events to come back."

Three of the teams in the Des Moines Regional had combined for 28 losses. Overall No. 1 seed Baylor had zero. Tennessee and Georgia Tech arrived in Iowa with identical records at 26–8, Kansas was 21–12, and Baylor was 36–0. The Lady Bears didn't feel any pressure with the perfect slate. "I don't think we've ever felt any pressure. We're honored to be here; we don't take things for granted," said Mulkey, who noted the 16 teams left in the tournament all share the same goal: win a national championship.

The Tennessee players said win-loss records lose significance in post-season. "We've had some losses that we shouldn't have had this season, and I am sure Kansas and Georgia Tech have probably had some as well," Massengale said. "Right now it comes down to who can play the best at game time." The Lady Vols had gone from one extreme to the other from the last game to the next as far as game time was concerned. The pre-game meal in Des Moines would be breakfast. "Can we get some happy medium like a 2 o'clock tip?" Mickie DeMoss said with a smile. "If I had to choose between the two, I would rather go early because you are not sitting around all day."

Curfew is usually around 11 p.m. on the road, but it was moved up an hour the evening before the game with Kansas, and the players' phones were taken overnight to ensure they could get some rest and were not awakened by callers or text messages. "We're excited, ESPN, early morning game, chance to go to the Elite Eight so it just has a different demeanor," Massengale said. Neither Massengale nor Harrison is a morning person, but Taber Spani is very outgoing at dawn. "At six in the morning, I am like, 'Morning, guys!' and they are like, 'Taber . . . ,'" Spani said, drawing her name out slowly. Kamiko Williams, who grew up on or close to Army bases, was usually up with the sun. "That is our alarm clock," Meighan Simmons said.

The weather was wonderful all day that Saturday. It was unseasonably warm in Des Moines with temperatures in the 70s. Wells Fargo Arena did have a sign for the tornado evacuation route, but that didn't come into play for the Lady Vols in this postseason tournament. In fact, the weather helped pre-sales with about 7,000 tickets sold in advance. "You can walk outside with normal clothes on," DeMoss said. "You're not bundled up. Chicago was beautiful. We come here. It's beautiful. I talked to some friends down in the Panhandle and they're like, 'It's going to rain all day.' I said, 'Well, it's beautiful in Des Moines, Iowa.' We've gotten real lucky with the weather."

The Lady Vols took survive and advance a little too seriously in the March 24 semifinal against Kansas. The Jayhawks opened the game by attacking the basket and got to the rim against the Lady Vols whether they were in man or zone defenses. "Our defense was awful, so we were stressing defending one-on-one, getting back and matching up, talking, getting stops, getting rebounds," Holly Warlick said. "We just were not very good in the first 15 minutes of the game."

The Lady Vols buried themselves in a hole, and freshman Ariel Massengale and sophomore Meighan Simmons came off the bench to get Tennessee out of the ditch. They jump-started the offense and played their best defense of the season. Still, the first half belonged to Kansas as the Jayhawks, led by point guard Angel Goodrich, got to the paint at will. "We want to be the ones to attack, and we did," Goodrich said. She had 12 points and three assists by the break. If Goodrich wasn't scoring, she was finding an open teammate. "She did about whatever she wanted to do," Warlick said. "She's difficult to defend because she shoots the long three, she penetrates, and she's a great passer. We tried trapping; she went under the screen and she hit a three. We tried switching, and she went around."

Tennessee took an early 2–0 lead when Glory Johnson drove and dished the ball to Vicki Baugh, but Kansas took the lead on back-to-back layups by Chelsea Gardner and built it to 14 points, 26–12, on a jumper from Aishah Sutherland, "You've got to stay poised, and you've got to have confidence," said Alicia Manning, who hit a baseline jumper early in the game. "We knew we weren't playing our best basketball, and our best was yet to come. And then it came, and that is how we turned the game around." Taber Spani got the rally started with a three ball, and then Massengale found Shekinna Stricklen in transition. But Spani tweaked her knee on defense—she said she felt a shift—and had to seek Jenny Moshak on the sideline. She looked visibly uncomfortable after the incident and plunged her legs into an ice bath immediately after the game. But Spani wasn't the only one with discomfort; Stricklen left the game to get treated for leg cramps, and Baugh, who has issues with tight hamstrings, had trouble getting and staying loose. "It happened in both of my legs," Baugh said. "They tighten up and lock on me, and it's very hard to straighten my leg out."

Simmons played lockdown defense, boxed out, got the rebound and then hit a three on the other end to trim the lead to 28–20 with 7:04 to play before the break. Dean Lockwood heaped high praise on Simmons after the game. "Her on-ball defense was tremendous. I got fired up watching that kid guard Kansas on the perimeter." The coaching staff challenged the entire team. "Are you just on defense or are you really playing defense?" Lockwood said. "I think early we were just on defense. We started to really play defense. They hurt us on ball screens and flare screens. We got a lot more determined. That is what defense is. You had better be determined to play through actions and you're going to get hit with screens. But instead of dying on the first action, you've got to have multiple efforts."

Simmons missed on the next trey ball, but Johnson got the rebound and stick-back to cut the lead to 28–22, and Kansas Coach Bonnie Henrickson called timeout at the 6:30 mark. "There are lots of different ways those guys can score," Henrickson said. The Lady Vols didn't completely wipe out Kansas' lead in the game's first 20 minutes, but Johnson hit a turn-around in the paint, and Stricklen made one of two free throws to go into the locker down by just five points, 35–30. "We had a pretty heated discussion at halftime," Warlick said. "Our program is built on defense and rebounds, and we were not doing that. We had to get down and defend one-on-one, and I thought we came out and did that."

The players said the discussion started among themselves before the coaches even spoke to them. Aishah Sutherland hit a jumper for Kansas to start the second half, and then the Lady Vols went to work. Massengale pulled Tennessee to within one and then tied the game at 42 with back-to-back three pointers and 16:28 left to play. "It was now or never," Massengale said. "We just took it one possession at a time." Five minutes into the second half, Johnson gave the Lady Vols the lead with a short jumper. The crowd of 7,941—the majority wearing orange—roared its approval, and Tennessee's post players stayed in attack mode.

Baugh was fouled at the rim and made the first free throw but missed the second. Johnson snared the offensive board, got fouled, and hit both from the stripe to give the Lady Vols a 47–44 lead with 13:33 left. When Massengale connected on a jumper for a 49–44 lead with 12:30 left, Henrickson called for a timeout. Goodrich responded with a jumper, but then Tennessee's defense stiffened—Stricklen got a block—and the offense got in running gear. Simmons got to the rim, and Kamiko Williams entered the game and did the same thing. "A lot of it honestly came from Briana," Williams said when asked about her effective play in the second half. "She gets on me all the time. She calls me lazy and I don't do this or that, so a couple of minutes before I got in there she said, 'Be ready, be ready.' While I'm in there playing I can hear her on the bench yelling, 'Good job, Kamiko! Do this and do that.'"

Johnson got fouled and hit her free throws, and Baugh got an offensive board and hit a nifty reverse for a 61–53 lead with 7:32 left. "Obviously their speed in transition got the best of us," Henrickson said. A steal by Massengale led to the next basket as she got the ball ahead to Williams, who found Simmons for the layup—a 63–53 lead with 7:07 to play and another Kansas timeout. But the Lady Vols kept attacking. Johnson got a defensive board and got the ball to Baugh, who passed ahead to Williams, who again connected with Simmons for a layup and a 67–55 lead. That was followed by a Simmons steal, a layup, and a 69–55 lead with 5:58 left.

Tennessee kept the lead in double digits, twice reaching 16 points, but Kansas fought until the final buzzer. The Jayhawks could not, however, keep the Lady Vols off the glass, and then they had to foul. Massengale hit four free throws, and Johnson connected on two for the final 84–73 score. Goodrich led Kansas with 23 points, Sutherland tallied 19, Chelsea Gardner added 14, and Monica Engelman chipped in with eight. Meanwhile Simmons led Tennessee with 22 points, an NCAA tourney high for the sophomore, and three other players reached double digits with Johnson at 18 points, Stricklen at 16, and Massengale at 12. Tennessee had 15 assists, just eight turnovers, six steals, and a block. The Lady Vols prevailed on the boards, 41–32. Baugh had a game-high 11 rebounds, while Stricklen grabbed nine and Johnson had seven. That brought Johnson's career total to 1,204, and she became the second Lady Vol in program history to tally more than 1,200 rebounds (the first was Chamique Holdsclaw). Johnson also moved into the 13th spot on the career scoring list with 1,624 points, passing Dana Johnson.

Tennessee outpaced Kansas in second-chance points, 23–12, while the paint scoring was almost even: 46 for Kansas, 45 for Tennessee. The Lady Vol bench outscored its counterpart, 41–11. It was truly a tale of two halves for Tennessee. The Lady Vols scored 30 in the first and 54 in the second. They shot 36.4 percent before halftime and 51.5 percent afterwards. "We didn't start out well at all, but the second half was definitely a different half for us," Pat Summitt said. Simmons scored 16 points in the second half, and all of Massengale's points came after halftime. "Glory, Alicia Manning, and Vicki Baugh came in at halftime and said, 'You need to shoot the ball. We need you to be a part of the offense,'" Massengale said. "They had confidence in me, and I just had to go out there and have enough confidence in myself to knock down those shots for this team."

The Lady Vols reached the program's 25th Elite Eight. The season had been about the Tennessee seniors trying to reach their first Final Four, but it was the underclassmen that provided the boost in Des Moines in the semifinal. They would all have their hands full Monday against Baylor, which won easily against Georgia Tech (83–68) and whose theme was "Unfinished Business" after a loss in the Elite Eight in 2011. The Lady Vols would face Brittney Griner, who electrified the crowd at Wells Fargo Arena with a two-handed slam against Georgia Tech that even got Tennessee fans off their feet to applaud.

"We're both trying to get to a Final Four," Baylor Coach Kim Mulkey said. "She has seniors who haven't been, and we have a kid who's supposed to be the greatest post player to play the game who's never won a championship." The Lady Bears showed signs of weakness in that 2011 tourney, but that wasn't the case in 2012. The score against Georgia Tech wasn't indicative of Baylor's dominance, as the Lady Bears led by 31 points and then made wholesale substitutions with six minutes left. The game against Georgia Tech was essentially over midway through the first half.

To get to Baylor, the Lady Vols had to take care of Kansas, and they did so with a come-from-behind win. Henrickson took a moment in the post-game handshake line to lean in and speak to Summitt. "'I've always had great respect for you, and I always will,'" Henrickson said when asked what she said to Summitt. "It's not just that she's won all those games, which is amazing to me; it's how she's handled success and all of that—just who she is as a person and how she's handled her situation. I wanted to make sure I told her when I got a chance."

33

ELITE EIGHT

wo teams remained in Des Moines, and they sat down with the media the day before they met on a Monday night for a berth at the Final Four in Denver. While the focus was basketball, the topics can veer off the court, which is how the latest dance craze became known as the Dean Lockwood.

Both Tennessee and Baylor reached this point in 2011 and fell short, Tennessee to Notre Dame and Baylor to Texas A&M. The Lady Vol seniors were seeking their first Final Four, and somehow they had to not let how much they wanted to reach it interfere with the effort it would take to do so. For Glory Johnson, that meant zeroing in on basketball and the matchup instead of the ramifications of the outcome. "Stay focused and take advantage of the scouting report that the coaches give us," Johnson said. "They give it to us with enough time to study it and know our personnel. Go into the game feeling comfortable, feeling relaxed and with confidence."

Coach Pat Summitt had sometimes used the expression: "Be careful what you show me." Kamiko Williams nodded and smiled in the locker room when a puzzled Ariel Massengale and Meighan Simmons were asked about it. It was then explained to them that the defense they played against Kansas—and in Simmons' case her board play, too—would now be expected every outing. When a player showed Summitt what she could do, the head coach knew the player was indeed capable. "Yep, yep," Williams said with a laugh as Massengale and Simmons got wide-eyed, recognizing how their performance would impact the staff's expectations going forward.

"Ohhhh," Massengale said. Defense and rebounding are as much about heart as they are about footwork and position, and Tennessee needed that same level of desire from Simmons and Massengale if the Lady Vols were to reach a goal that had been lying just beneath the surface all season. "I have to be consistent," Simmons said. "I think it's a matter of me making sure I have that mindset to go out there and play and use these past games to say, 'You know what? If I can do it then, why can't I do it again?' " Massengale had started her Lady Vol career playing well on the defensive end and then dipped as the season continued. "It might have been fatigue; the college season is long," Massengale said. "The SEC is a tough conference to play in. There are some great guards in this conference." The postseason had been about the seniors, but Johnson said the veterans have embraced the underclassmen. "We need the baby ones," Johnson said.

"Awwww," Massengale said. "We can't do it by ourselves. If they're willing to go to bat for us, then we are willing to work as hard as we can for them."

Tennessee entered the game as the undisputed underdog, a role the Lady Vols were not accustomed to playing in the NCAA postseason. The Lady Vols have had considerable NCAA success in Iowa and were 7–1 in postseason games in the Hawkeye State. The current team was aware of the history, thanks to Debby Jennings, the longtime media relations chief for the Lady Vols. "Debby Jennings keeps a great record of everything," Taber Spani said. "I think she probably memorizes every single fact in Lady Vol history, so we are aware of that, and it is pretty interesting."

Both teams felt considerable pressure to succeed, especially after coming up short at this same slot in the tourney bracket a year ago. Baylor went to a Final Four when Brittney Griner was a freshman. The only player to experience that for Tennessee was graduate Vicki Baugh, a fifth-year redshirt after two ACL surgeries. "I think, in addition to doing this for Pat Summitt, these five seniors have something to prove, not only for the Tennessee tradition but also for themselves," Holly Warlick said. "They are probably one of the hardest working teams we have had. They have been thrown a lot of curves, and for the most part, they have handled it. I keep saying their best basketball is yet to come. Let's hope it comes on Monday night and keeps getting better."

When she wasn't on the court, Briana Bass was very vocal on the bench. She played the part of coach and motivator. "I think over the years, not being able to play as much and trying to find my way on this team and how I could contribute, I came up with encouragement and trying to be like a coach," Bass said. Williams is a physically gifted 5'11" guard who didn't always play to her capability in college, though she did so as a senior during the 2012–13 season. Bass didn't mince words with the junior and gave Williams an earful during the Kansas game. "I told Miko that she needed to be focused here in the mind and that we really needed her, and we needed her heart. She went in there and played her butt off."

Johnson had a better shot at getting a board if the guards did their part, too. If perimeter players didn't box out, then Johnson had to fend off the opposing post and the guard darting in who was left unchecked. Johnson delivered specific instructions during the Kansas game to Simmons to make sure she boxed out her player. Apparently Johnson was a tad more emphatic that Saturday, and Simmons responded with four rebounds. Simmons also boxed out, which helped the post players immensely: it kept the guards from slipping underneath them (they sometimes fouled, but officials tended not to call it and instead sided with the smaller player over the bigger one), and it also helped eliminate long rebounds that start fast breaks for the opposing team. "The long rebounds, we're all in the paint, so it's up to the guards to get it," Johnson said. "And if the guards don't get it, they're already running down the floor, and we're behind them. It's really hard if the guards don't rebound." It was also why Shekinna Stricklen played extended minutes, even if she was struggling with her shot. Stricklen was consistently on the glass, and Simmons also responded in Iowa. "I think she was tired of me yelling at her," Johnson said, while Simmons burst out with laughter. "It worked." Former Lady Vol Alex Fuller used to tell teammates: "Just find somebody and hit 'em."

"Yep, and it works," Johnson said.

The players stayed loose in the locker room, which was important with the weight of an Elite Eight game. The always-enthusiastic Lockwood inspired the "Dean Lockwood dance," which Bass and Isabelle Harrison demonstrated for the media. It involved sliding in the paint, backing up to box out, and getting arms in the air, accompanied by common Lockwood instructions. Lockwood was in tears laughing while he watched the live version in the locker room, and it was a great moment for a team that had been asked for seven months about Summitt and her future as the Lady Vols'

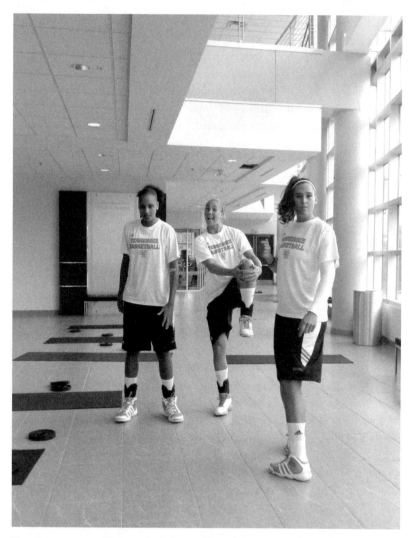

The players managed to keep their sense of humor that season. From left, Cierra Burdick, Alicia Manning, and Taber Spani react to the camera.

head coach. "Basically, we just try to stay in the present," Alicia Manning said. "Whatever Coach Summitt decides to do after this, we support her. We have had her back this whole season. She is such a great person and is going to leave her legacy whether it is this year, next year, five years down the road, 10 years down the road."

If Baylor's perfect run was to be derailed, a team would have to get baskets from the outside. Tennessee did so to open the game—the senior lineup did its job—and had a 9–4 lead at the first media timeout after Vicki Baugh drove and kicked back to Shekinna Stricklen, who drained the three-pointer. For Tennessee to do well, Stricklen, Johnson, and Baugh had to play well. And they were ready for the opening tip. "They are kind of like the lead horses," Lockwood said. "When the lead horses are working and you see the snow flying, everybody else is coming." But then Baylor got hot, and Tennessee went cold. Baylor took the lead at the 12:48 mark of the first half, and the Lady Vols were in catch-up mode the rest of the way. "I said it before the game: It goes further than Brittney Griner," Holly Warlick said. "They all play well together, and they were exceptional. We look at what they did offensively, but they're outstanding on the defensive end. They force you to take quick shots. They're just a great basketball team."

Baylor's defensive pressure had improved, as the guards were stickier on the shooters than in the first matchup last November in Knoxville, a game the Lady Vols nearly won. They applied tight pressure, because Brittney Griner roamed around the paint and its edges and erased mistakes with blocks and altered shots. Tennessee knew that to have success against Baylor it would need to manage Griner, take care of the ball, and hit shots from the perimeter. The Lady Vols managed to do two of the three. Tennessee had just 11 turnovers total—only four in the second half—and bottled up Griner in the first half, but the Lady Vols shot 11.1 percent (1–9) from the arc before halftime. Tennessee collapsed the paint around Griner and held the 6'8" post to a 3–10 shooting stat in the first half, but Baylor guards Odyssey Sims and Kimetria Hayden shot 5–8 from the arc before halftime, and Tennessee was in a 35–20 hole at the break.

The long ball didn't get any better after the break. The Lady Vols were 3–12 from long range in the second half and shot 19.0 percent for the game from the arc. Baylor, meanwhile, connected at 53.3 percent from long range, and Griner got on track in the second half—she was 5–8 from the field after halftime. The Lady Vols made several stabs at a comeback in the second half. Tennessee cut a 15-point deficit to nine points, 35–26, at the 17:58 mark after Baugh found Johnson inside, Manning hit a baseline jumper, and Stricklen found Baugh inside. Mulkey called timeout, and Sims hit a three on Baylor's next possession to extend the lead back to double digits. The Lady Vols trimmed it to eight, 44–36, on a catch-and-shoot stick-back by Isabelle Harrison with 12:43 to play and again on a layup by Stricklen, 46–38, with 11:39 to play. Again Sims stuck a three to boost it back to double digits.

"Our defense broke down a few times on their guards," Mickie DeMoss said. "We were so consumed with Griner. I thought we let Odyssey Sims get loose on us, Hayden a few times in the first half, so that kind of separated them. They made it tough on us to get good looks. We got some good looks, but we were shooting threes three steps behind the three-point line." The Lady Bears, led by Griner, had a player that no college team could match in terms of shot-blocking dominance and the ability to finish on the offensive end and play above the rim. "They're not going to invent a new defense to guard Griner, so I figured we'd see them sagging in the paint, zone, challenge us to shoot the perimeter shot," Baylor Coach Kim Mulkey said. "Nae-Nae (Hayden), Jordan (Madden), and Odyssey have done it time and time again. They can shoot it. Our offense flows and goes through Brittney Griner, but if you're going to leave us open we have to take that shot."

A trey by Stricklen and layup by Ariel Massengale fueled one last Tennessee run when the Lady Vols cut the lead to 64–53 with 4:50 to play, but Baylor answered on its end. Scoring in the game was completed with 2:20 left when Griner completed a three-point play at the foul line for the final 77–58 score. Griner, Madden, and Terran Condrey were not around for the final 46 seconds of the game after Sims missed two layups and ended up on the floor. Stricklen went to help her up, but she was standing over Sims, who took it another way and brushed away Stricklen's offer. The two players then engaged in a verbal discussion, with Cierra Burdick wrapping up Stricklen and pushing her away. "We got caught in the heat of the moment," Sims said. "We both just got a little rattled. That's it." Stricklen, who played USA ball with the fiery Sims, wasn't surprised at the reaction. "Not at all," Stricklen said. "I know her attitude. If you watched me play the four years that I've been here, you know I'm not that type of person," she continued. "I tripped, I tried to catch myself, I tried to help her up, and she just took it the wrong way. We just started talking back and forth to each other."

Three Baylor players left the bench and were ejected from the game. Lady Vols Vicki Baugh and Alicia Manning also left the bench, but the officials didn't see them and apparently they didn't appear on the TV footage reviewed at the scorer's table. A statement issued by official Bryan Enterline through a pool reporter stated that Griner, Madden, and Condrey were ejected for leaving the bench area. Double technical fouls were called on Sims and Stricklen, which offset the need for any free throws. "A bench technical foul should have been assessed regardless of the number of players that left the bench," Enterline stated. The incident occurred directly in front of Baylor's bench, and Manning and Baugh both said they saw Baylor's players on the court and reacted. "I saw their bench clear, and I wasn't about to leave Strick out there to dry so me and Vicki came in there to help her out. Nothing really happened, but we have each other's back no matter what happens," Manning said. Baugh added, "I didn't know what happened. I looked up and saw some people jump off the Baylor bench, so I was just going in there to have my teammate's back."

There also was an incident in the first half in which Johnson was fouled at the 4:23 mark and landed hard on her hip. She said the pain shot down her leg, and she needed assistance to leave the court. A trio at the end of Baylor's bench, two in warmups and another in street clothes, yelled at Johnson while she was down. Johnson returned to the bench with about a minute left to play in the first half and took the court for the start of the second half. "I can't leave my teammates out to dry, no matter what the pain is," Johnson said. "A game like this, you can't sit out."

The final two minutes featured missed shots by both teams, the confrontation between Stricklen and Sims, and a lengthy delay to review the courtside monitor before ejecting the three Baylor players who left the bench. Sims led Baylor with 27 points; Griner tallied 23 points, 15 boards, and nine blocks, while Hayden added 18 points. The trio accounted for 68 of Baylor's 77 points. Stricklen, who tallied 22 points and 11 boards, led Tennessee, while Johnson had 19 points and 14 rebounds, giving her 1,218 boards for her career, the second-best mark in Lady Vol program history. The teams were knotted on the glass at 47 rebounds each, a testament to the glass work of the Lady Vols, especially Johnson.

The Lady Vol seniors became the first class not to make a Final Four, but they also had the misfortune in timing to twice have to face Baylor in the postseason. Tennessee headed to the locker room while the Lady Bears trimmed the net and celebrated the Final Four berth.

On March 26, 2012, Pat Summitt coached her final game for the Lady Vols.

34

THE FINAL POST-GAME

The crowd at Wells Fargo Arena was already on its feet—the Baylor fans were celebrating the win and Tennessee fans were saluting Pat Summitt. As Summitt made her way through the handshake line and off the court, photographers followed her every step, as the end of an incredible era in all of sports unfolded in front of them.

Mickie DeMoss, who had been with Summitt for so many years and was headed to the sideline of the WNBA's Indiana Fever, knew it was her final walk with the head coach. DeMoss' plans to exit college and head to the pro ranks had been set in motion around midseason. "She was the primary reason that I came back to Tennessee," DeMoss said. "I just felt like it would be hard, too many facets to staying without her there. It was time for Holly to staff her own program. It was time for me to move on and let some new blood come in there. The Fever situation just happened to pop up as all this was going on. It kind of fell into my lap.

"The whole year . . . I can't sit here and say that I was walking off going, oh yeah, how traumatic this is and this is our last game. It was the whole year of processing it. It was difficult, but there were a lot of games that were difficult. I don't think I looked at it as, 'This is the end.' Maybe that was just my way of not wanting to think that. I don't have any specific memories of that last game . . . I think it was all year that I was processing it. It happened quite a bit throughout the year."

The full weight of the season descended upon the players and staff as they headed to the back hallways of the arena and toward their locker room. Lockwood had been on autopilot since August 2011, refusing to break down. As he made his way with the team to the locker room, the emotional unraveling began. "Honestly, I didn't until the end. In my quiet moments, there was sadness, but I was so . . . We have a job to do it. There is a real need for all of us to hold this together for Pat, for this program. I can't afford the luxury of breaking down. I was so consumed. There was a long race to run. We can't afford to feel sorry for ourselves. It's not about how I feel. It's about what we need to do. It's about this mission. Once the mission ended, then it became more emotional for me."

Lockwood's eyes reddened and his voice shook as he recounted that walk in Des Moines. He found an analogy, this time the Clint Eastwood movie, *Hang 'Em High*. Eastwood plays the role of Jed Cooper, who is seeking to bring some men to justice under harrowing and exhausting circumstances. "He's riding into town and he's conscious but it takes so much out of him that as soon as he's coming into town, he just falls off his horse," Lockwood said. "That is how it felt."

It was an emotional night for the Lady Vols and its coaching staff. As Warlick left the locker room with Glory Johnson and Shekinna Stricklen, who were in tears, she wrapped an arm around each player. Warlick also got emotional during the post-game press conference. "This team is about Pat Summitt, and this team has battled all year," Warlick told the media. "I'm proud of them. I think, like Pat, this team never gave up." Warlick's post-game tears weren't over the loss of a game; "Oh, Lord no," Warlick said.

She also felt the weight of the season with every step in the behind-the-scenes area of Wells Fargo Arena and especially as she walked into the locker room. "You walk back there, and you see these kids crying. And you're like, 'This is it. It really is.' I think I realized it when I went to the press conference. I cried at the press conference." Summitt spoke to the team during the cooling-off time period. "She said, 'Get your heads up. I love y'all,'" Warlick said.

But the players could not stop their tears.

"I had never seen Vicki cry. I had never seen Glory cry," Meighan Simmons said. "Just to see so many emotions . . . walking off the floor, you want to think about what you didn't do or what you did do but at that one particular moment the emotions were so heavy, so, so heavy, that to the point when you walked into the hallway, silence. You couldn't say anything. All you could hear is shoes walking across the floor. Of course you could hear Baylor cheering, but when we got to our side, silence. I think everybody knew deep down that that was Pat's last time. We got into the locker room, and it was worse. It felt like a loud rainstorm. Everybody was crying. I didn't cry until I got in there. And when she got up to speak it was just like whoa, what in the world. I will never forget that feeling because from her speaking and her being the first person to come up and say something, I knew right there. I said to myself, 'This is probably going to be her last time. Take in every moment.' I think everybody took her in and embraced her at that moment."

"I remember her telling us that she loved us," Vicki Baugh said. "A lot of it didn't have to do with basketball, and I respect that a lot. I think hearing her final words, we knew what we could do. Pat knew what we could do. This was a mother talking to her girls. It had nothing to do with the Xs and Os. It was about being a woman and growing as a woman." It was quintessential Summitt that she didn't make her final post-game talk about her. Simmons was correct. The proverbial writing was on the wall, and Summitt later said in an affidavit that Athletics Director Dave Hart told her before the 2012 NCAA tourney began that the season would be her last, a meeting Summitt characterized as "surprising" and "hurtful." The Tennessee administration disputed her account, calling it a misunderstanding of the conversation, but nearly everyone in that locker room thought this was it for Summitt.

Johnson was inconsolable. Not only was her career over without a Final Four, but she was also saying goodbye to Summitt. Media cameras later showed Summitt comforting her crying senior. "I tried my hardest to get us there," Johnson said of the Final Four. "I know I tried everything I could. It was very, very tough. She knew we were trying to do everything that we could. I was trying to put everything out there on the floor." Johnson's emotional spiral started before the clock hit zero on the game. "It was so tough. A couple of us went down before the game was even over, breaking down on the court, just knowing this was going to be her last game and nothing would ever be the same," Johnson said. "And we lost, so it was just making it worse. We all broke down, and we were able to find comfort with Pat. She told us that she was proud of each and every one of us."

The players weren't the only ones crying; the support staff was overcome with emotion, too. "We were shedding tears," Jenny Moshak said. "The tears could have been assumed that they were associated with the loss, but it was more than just the loss. And then the hugs started before even getting to the locker room. We knew it was the end of something very special. The finality. Going out that hard. It was so exhausting at that point. It was entirely exhausting. Before the game you knew they were going to fight . . . they had left everything. By the end, there was nothing left in the tank. They were trying to full throttle it. The weight of the world was on them."

"First of all, everyone was upset and emotional about losing an Elite Eight game," Taber Spani said. "We had done it for the second year in a row. Everyone is totally heartbroken over that, but everyone was thinking, 'Was that Pat's last go-around? Was that her last time?' I remember her saying how proud she was of our team. Everyone was kind of losing it in their own way. The seniors talked. It was a special time, but it was a time you wanted to hold onto for as long as possible. You hold onto those memories and not let it slip away."

"It was tough without question because that was it, and for her it's too soon to be it. It was tough to see," said Meshia Thomas, who, as always, was near Summitt. "It wasn't about the loss to me. It was about the loss to the sport. It was about her. Such an incredible icon. Such an incredible mentor. Well respected. Revered by so many. It was tough to see this giant, this gentle giant . . . that was it."

Lockwood will always remember that Summitt, to the end, stayed in the moment. "It wasn't about Pat. Even listening to her that day, it wasn't reflective. It wasn't what an honor it's been to be here. It wasn't a sendoff message," Lockwood said. "It was an end of the season message. I remember she said, 'To be honest with you, losing just flat out sucks.' I remember that so clearly. 'There is nothing I can tell you that's going to change that. Losing sucks.' She told them she was proud of them. The wheels are really turning. Are we seeing her last post-game speech here? None of us really knew for sure, but we had an inkling that things could go that way. If this were me, I might get more reflective, but Pat is so in the moment of dealing with this game, this team, here and now. Glory got up and gave her a big hug. And other players spoke up and thanked Pat."

Spani will always remember the emotion that coursed through that locker room. The season had felt like a farewell tour, and the finality washed over the players and staff. "It was a culmination of the entire year," Spani said. "We were hoping it would not be her last game, but every away game we went to that season, she was getting standing ovations. It was like the last go-around. Everyone can celebrate her while she's still head coach. I felt like that everywhere we went, everyone was always paying their respects to who she is."

After the cooling-off period, standard after all athletic events, the media was allowed inside the locker room, where players were huddled in their lockers with red eyes and tears still flowing. Spani was nearly inconsolable, but she handled the interviews. "We battled, and we're proud of that," Spani said. "We never gave up until the final buzzer. It hurts no matter what, but it just really hurts for these seniors. It hurts not to do it for that senior class and for Coach. That really hurts. Our coaches and everyone in here said they (the seniors) can't hang their heads because they battled. They battled so hard."

Ariel Massengale had her head buried in her hands, as did Kamiko Williams, but both were able to speak about the game. "It hurts bad," Massengale said. "Today we had the opportunity to make it to the Final Four and it didn't happen. But Tennessee is still one of the best programs in the country, and we've just got to get back to work." Massengale said the players discussed at halftime that they were getting good looks but needed those shots to fall. "But all credit to Baylor," Massengale said. "They played their game plan to a T. They played hard and got after it. We just couldn't hit shots when we needed to."

Tennessee also had issues with foul trouble. Baugh had four fouls, and Isabelle Harrison fouled out in six minutes of play. "It really hurt when Vick got into foul trouble," Stricklen said. "But she held her ground. Izzy came in, and she held her ground. This team, I love it, we fought. I think we started out focusing too much on Griner. They were getting open threes. I give them a lot of credit. They were knocking down shots and some shots weren't falling for us." Stricklen got emotional when asked about the end of her career. "I learned a lot these four years that is going to help me in life, in the real world, not just in basketball," Stricklen said. "Playing under the best coach, she teaches you for life."

Baugh shed tears in her locker while trying to wrap up the five years she spent at Tennessee. She left with a national title ring from 2008. "I have no regrets of anything that happened," Baugh said. "We played a hard basketball game against one of the best teams that I've played in my career. I am extremely proud of this team and how we pulled together. It's not over for Tennessee. We're still going to get a lot better. I am just looking forward to being able to watch and continue to support the program."

The staff saluted the seniors after the game in recognition of their efforts, especially to reach the Elite Eight and then to battle throughout the game. "They put us in a position to get to a Final Four two years in a row," DeMoss said. "There are eight teams left playing, and we were one of them. We know our standards are very high at Tennessee, but it wasn't a lack of effort." The seniors didn't make a Final Four, but that is not how they should be remembered. They absorbed countless blows on and off the court—none more gut-wrenching than Summitt's diagnosis—and they stayed on their feet.

Baugh returned for a fifth season after recovering from three knee surgeries. The four true seniors endured one of the worst seasons in Lady Vol history when they were thrust into roles as freshmen that they weren't ready for because of graduation and injuries. They survived Summitt's wrath and Heather Mason's boot camp after the 2009 season, responding with double SEC titles, regular season and tourney, the following season. All five seniors wore the academic excellence torch patches on their jerseys, and three graduated early and pursued master's degrees in their final year. The other two graduated on time. "They did a lot," DeMoss said. "They've been great leaders for these young kids, particularly this year. Pat told them how much she appreciated everything they've done and how they've represented Tennessee."

Summitt stayed in the coaches' room while the media was in the locker room, and when the door swung open, she could be seen sitting at a table talking to others in the room. Summitt comforted them, including *The New York Times* reporter Jere Longman, who asked to speak with Summitt so he could thank her for all she did for the sport. "The thing about Mom is it was always about others," Tyler Summitt said. "It was always about relationships, and it was always about love. It was very emotional, but there was a lot of love."

After the media left, it was time for the players and coaches to prepare for departure. A bus took them to the airport for a chartered flight back to Knoxville. Tyler stayed by his mother's side after the final horn sounded. "I walked with her from the court to the locker room. I stayed in the coaches' room, went out and watched her talk to the players and then went back in the coaches' room and then I walked with her to the bus. I was with her the whole time," Tyler said. "I don't think she was sad about it being her last game so much as she didn't like to lose. She was mad they lost and also missing the seniors and thinking about the seniors."

"Just seeing Pat walk out . . . she walked out with Tyler, and I was like, 'Wow, this is it,'" Thomas said. "I knew she wasn't going to be back. It wasn't fair to her to put her in that situation."

Summitt made her way to the bus, which still had to be loaded with gear, and waited for the players and staff to join her. As always, a crowd had gathered. Summitt could have left in a private car. She could have sought privacy at a crushing personal and professional time. But she saw the autograph seekers and well-wishers and stood up. "There were people outside. She got off the bus twice to sign autographs," Thomas said. "I don't even really know if it hits her that she truly is what she is. If I could bottle that grace in a jar and take it myself, I would want that. She is the queen of what she does. I feel honored to have walked alongside her."

35

EVE OF ANNOUNCEMENT

The voice on the other end of the phone didn't sound at all like Pat Summitt's. But it was. It was the eve of her press conference to officially announce her retirement, and Summitt was crying.

Earlier that same day on April 18, 2012, Summitt had made phone calls to three sportswriters: Sally Jenkins of *The Washington Post*, Dan Fleser of the *Knoxville News Sentinel*, and me. She wanted that trio to hear the news from her before the public announcement and allow the writers to publish stories on their respective websites before it broke nationally. She sounded upbeat as she discussed her reasons for stepping down and accepting the role as head coach emeritus. Holly Warlick was officially introduced as the new head coach on April 19, 2012, a decision embraced by Lady Vol Nation.

Warlick, who had been at Summitt's side since 1985, took over the program after an emotionally wrenching season. A Knoxville native and Lady Vol point guard from 1976–80, she handled dual roles when Summitt had to curtail her daily activities due to her diagnosis. Summitt had opted to return to coach for that final 2011–12 season with her assistants absorbing additional daily duties, none more so than Warlick. Summitt endorsed the plan of having Warlick succeed her at Tennessee. "I am excited for her," Summitt said. "I think I can help her and obviously she is going to be there for me. We are going to keep on keeping on."

Summitt remained with the program and was still part of practice planning and meetings with players, especially during the 2012–13 season. As she focused more on her health, however, Summitt's regular involvement decreased. Tennessee had consulted beforehand with the NCAA to determine precisely the parameters of Summitt's duties. "We haven't outlined everything," Summitt said the day before the official retirement press conference. "I know that these players are going to need us. We lost five seniors. I want to do all I can to help Holly. I am trying to get some great players in here."

The decision for Summitt developed over the course of the season. She knew the illness had diminished her in some ways in terms of the energy and daily commitment it takes to be the head of Lady Vols basketball, but she also knew that she still had plenty to offer to the players. It was a difficult conclusion for Summitt to reach. "I felt like after my diagnosis I was doing less and less," Summitt said. "I was just trying to figure out where my next place was going to be, and rather than stay on as a head coach, Holly and I talked. She is going to need me, and I am going to need her so I feel really good about it." Warlick chose the new assistant coaches with input from Summitt, who would no longer sit on the bench during games. Assistant Coach Dean Lockwood remained on the staff, and he was a critical connection to several 2013 recruiting targets.

Recruiting always enters a critical cycle in April because it marks the beginning of showcase events for top high school talent. Summitt knew she had to bring clarity to the coaching situation at Tennessee for the sake of recruiting. Rival schools and recruiting services with agendas to steer their players to certain colleges were using Summitt's illness against Tennessee.

April 18, 2012, is a momentous date in Lady Vol history because Summitt—a coach who started her career at age 22 while teaching classes at Tennessee and working on her master's degree—made public what had been anticipated. "I am good," Summitt said during the telephone interview. "I knew that this was going to be something that I would have to make a decision on, and I am happy about it. Holly has been doing an awful lot. She has really stepped up. She knows I am going to be there for her. We're going to keep on going. I'll be all over the place. Everything that they're going to let me do, I am going to do."

Summitt's exit as head coach meant that for the first time since 1974, Tennessee would open a basketball season with a new head coach on the bench for the Lady Vols. But Summitt promised to stick around. "I am not going anywhere. They are going to have to put up with me anyway," Summitt said. Those remarks were delivered with a laugh, an indication Summitt had made peace with the directive to retire but still remain close to the program. "I think it's important for the players. Some of them came here because of me and I just want them to know that I am not going anywhere. I will be there for them if they want to come in my office and talk. I am still going to be at Tennessee." That certainly was the case with Summitt's final signing class of Andraya Carter, Bashaara Graves, and Jasmine Jones. They came to Tennessee knowing that Summitt might not be on the sideline when they arrived.

Late in the afternoon on April 18, 2012, hours after talking to Summitt, I was waiting inside the newsroom of local television station, WATE-TV Channel 6. An hour-long special about Summitt was being aired, and I was asked to provide commentary. Carter had agreed to be interviewed on the air by telephone from her home in Flowery Branch, Georgia, near the end of the hour. I was placing a quick reminder call to Carter, but I accidentally hit Summitt's number when opening the call log on the phone. A voicemail greeting indicated the error, and since it was nearly time to go inside the studio, I ended that call and quickly called Carter to verify her availability and remind her to be ready during the show. During that exchange, Summitt had called back and left a voicemail, saying to call her if I needed anything. I placed a call to Summitt to explain the earlier error.

But Summitt sounded completely different than she had hours earlier during the phone interview with *InsideTennessee.* In fact, Summitt sounded emotional and her voice was barely audible at times. She was crying. I ducked into an empty office for privacy. When I asked Summitt whether she wanted to officially retire the next day, initially there was silence. I again asked, "Pat, is this what you really want to do?" When Summitt spoke, I could hear the anguish in her voice. Summitt said she didn't want to step down, but she knew she had to do so. She didn't want that said on television the day before her press conference—she wanted a smooth process, especially for Warlick's transition, because that was best for Tennessee. Summitt's voice cracked while she talked.

I had never heard Summitt cry and tried to offer some words of comfort. Summitt said she would be OK, and the conversation ended. I honored Summitt's request and didn't mention the tears during the televised special. But it was a conversation seared into memory.

Pat Summitt doesn't cry. She did on the last evening that she was officially the head coach of Tennessee.

36

END OF AN ERA

Pat Summitt needed a speech for her retirement ceremony, so she called
Debby Jennings, as she had so many times for media assistance over
the past 35 years. Jennings knew Summitt needed a memorable gesture,
not just words, to convey what was happening at Tennessee. The program
needed a powerful image that would both signal the transition and put
Holly Warlick at ease. Jennings had just a few hours to prepare Summitt's
statement in what would be her final press conference, and she provided
Summitt with the signature moment.

Summitt summoned Warlick to her spot on the stage—one erected just
in front of the logo that bears Summitt's name on the court—took her whistle
out of a pocket and placed it around the neck of her longtime assistant. With
that gesture, what had been known for 24 hours seemed official: Summitt
was stepping down as head coach at the University of Tennessee, and Warlick
was succeeding the legend she had played for and worked beside for 31 total
years. Summitt's son, Tyler, was at her side on the stage. Warlick's mother,
Fran Warlick, occupied a front row seat at the press conference.

It was an afternoon of announcements and anecdotes with the current Lady Vols sitting in one section, at times laughing and at other times wiping tears from their eyes. When a photomontage was displayed on the overhead video, one of the last images depicted Summitt and the five seniors on what was now her last team. Every member of the 2011–12 team was in attendance for the event, which was held at Thompson-Boling Arena. An overflow of media occupied the areas in front and to the sides of the stage, and multiple news outlets carried the press conference live. Summitt had a prepared statement that outlined her joy that on the same day she announced she was retiring, her son announced he had accepted a job as an assistant coach for the women's basketball program at Marquette. She also joked about her starting salary—$250 a month at a time when she was bouncing checks—and talked about growing up on a dairy farm and how that instilled in her the value of hard work.

Summitt saluted the 161 women who had worn orange for the Lady Vols and vowed to the players sitting in the front two rows to Summitt's left that she would always be available to them. "I can promise you ladies, I'm here for you," Summitt said. "Trust me, that will happen. The success of the Lady Vols will always, always continue." Summitt closed her speech with a message to the fans and asked Warlick to stand up. "Finally, I have a special message and challenge to our fans and our supporters," Summitt said. "You have helped to make Lady Vol Basketball very special. I need you right now—I want you to listen to this—to step up more than ever to support our new head coach. Holly, I want you to come up here. It is now time to turn over my whistle to you. Thank you." The mentor and pupil then embraced to applause and audible gasps as some attendees became emotional.

It was powerfully symbolic and also underscored the finality of what had just happened—that after 38 years Summitt would no longer be on the sideline as the head coach of the Lady Vol basketball program. She remained with the program as head coach emeritus with duties that included mentoring players, contacting recruits in basketball and other sports via email or handwritten notes, engaging in all on-campus activities with recruits, observing practice and analyzing the game with coaches, and assisting with the locker room enhancement project.

Summitt didn't just want to read her statement. She asked to be able to take media questions at the live press conference. The way she handled that session showed how capable she still was at that time. Summitt was asked what her top priority would be in her new role. "To come to work every day, to be around the student-athletes. Maybe they'll keep me young," the then-59-year-old Summitt said. "I'm getting ready to turn the big one but I can still, yeah, 30; hardly. But being around young people, it's a breath of fresh air every day. And having such a great group, our managers, everybody—they're invested, so they're still going to see me and I'm still going to yell at them. But I love these young people and, hopefully, they'll keep me young." It marked the end of a nearly four-decade era in women's college basketball, but Summitt's graciousness and sense of humor kept what could have been a sad day from being anything but for those in attendance. She made jokes, smiled at the videos and photomontage and wrapped her arm around Tyler and pointed to the screen when an image of him as a tyke at a net-cutting ceremony appeared.

Summitt handled the question-and-answer session with the media gracefully, as did Tyler. He had a catalogue on his computer of every basketball formation, offense and defense that he had ever encountered during various stints as a Lady Vols practice player and Vols walk-on. Tyler graduated from college and went on to work at Marquette as an assistant coach. He fielded questions about his new job the same day his mother ended a storied career and was asked to tell a story about an AAU team that he coached over the past weekend.

"We actually had five players," Tyler said, as his mother smiled beside him. "A lot of them were taking the ACT—I coach 17-and-under girls—they were taking the ACT. Academics first, right mom? They couldn't make the tournament, so I had five. One of them was actually late, and it's my policy that if you're late you're not going to start; you might not even play. So we started the game with four players. The refs, the other coach, and everybody in the stands were looking at me like I was crazy, but something my mom always instilled in me was that discipline comes first."

Those lessons deteriorated shortly thereafter. Just four years later on April 8, 2016, Tyler Summitt, who was married to his high school sweetheart, would resign as head coach of Louisiana Tech for having an inappropriate relationship with a player. The relationship had started at Marquette, and the player had transferred to Louisiana Tech when Tyler became the head coach in 2014. But on that day in 2012, the thought that Tyler Summitt would descend from grace so rapidly and in such damaging fashion would not have been fathomable. In hindsight, Tyler took on too much too soon from a wedding to college coaching. His mother's illness likely accelerated his timetable. He also was grieving what had happened to her and was trying to be the decision maker and caretaker when he needed to just be a son.

After Pat Summitt completed the Q&A portion of the live press conference, she departed with Mickey Dearstone, the Voice of the Lady Vols, for a radio session. That left Warlick on the stage to announce her elevation to head coach for the formal press conference. Oddly, Joan Cronan, the longtime women's athletics director, wasn't on the stage. She sat among the observers and other administrators. Dave Hart, vice chancellor and director of UT athletics, outlined his season-long observations that led him to select Warlick for the job. He pointed out the tough position that she was placed in and noted how well she had handled the role under unprecedented circumstances.

"Holly's name and Holly's presence on the bench are really woven into the fabric of Lady Vol basketball, but that is not why I made the decision to offer the job to Holly Warlick," Hart said. "That's nice, but that had nothing to do with that decision. Watching Holly perform this year in her role in a very unique circumstance with Pat fighting this terrible disease, watching Holly Warlick grow as a coach, as a person, and as someone who could handle the leadership role that was demanded—and that role went far beyond the norm as I indicated a moment ago.

"As the season progressed, I became more and more convinced that we did not need to go on a national search. Pat and I talked regularly as the season went along about a lot of things. There was a time late in the season when she said to me, 'Dave, if I made the decision, and I haven't made the decision yet, but if I made the decision not to coach next year, have you given any thought to who will follow?' And I said, 'I have, Pat. I am giving very serious consideration to Holly.' And she said, 'That would excite me.' And I don't think she said it, either, based on her being Holly's mentor or Holly being her former player. I think she made it very sincerely that she believed as I did, that Holly Warlick could perform in that role and perform very, very well."

There were invited guests at the press conference, along with family members, friends, and the team, and Warlick received sustained applause when Hart formally introduced her as the new head coach. The circumstances around Summitt's departure were in doubt, despite Hart's statement, because it didn't seem voluntary. The welcoming of Warlick, however, was never in doubt. She provided continuity to a team and incoming recruits that needed stability and a strong connection to Summitt.

"I feel like the luckiest person in the world," said Warlick, thanking Hart and UT Chancellor Jimmy Cheek, who both remained on stage with her. "I get to coach at a school that's always been in my blood, and this is my home.

It's only taken me 27 years to get to this point, and I just really didn't want to rush it. I told Pat to take all the time she needed." That brought laughter from the group and Warlick went on to explain why she stayed at Summitt's side for so long. "People have asked me, 'Why have you not left?' And I said, 'Why would I?' Why would I leave a place that is rich in tradition, has an unbelievable administration that has always supported women's basketball and women's sports, and has the most incredibly supportive fans in the country? It didn't take me being a genius to stay here and love what I do."

It was also announced that Assistant Coach Dean Lockwood would remain with the program. That provided much-needed continuity, especially since Lockwood was a critical recruiter of three players who turned out to be the signing class of 2013—Mercedes Russell, Jordan Reynolds, and Jannah Tucker. With the departure of Mickie DeMoss to the WNBA—ironically, she would later end up on Tyler Summitt's staff at Louisiana Tech—Warlick had two openings to fill. A few weeks later, former Lady Vol Kyra Elzy joined the staff, as did Jolette Law, the former head coach of Illinois. (DeMoss would join Nikki Caldwell's staff at LSU in 2016; Elzy would return to Kentucky's staff that same year.)

All three of Tennessee's 2012 recruits—Andraya Carter, Bashaara Graves, and Jasmine Jones—came to Knoxville as planned. "Draya is diehard Tennessee," Graves said. "I'm a diehard. Jasmine is, too. That is what it came down to. We're diehard Tennessee." All three players had held signing ceremonies at their high schools in November 2011. Graves signed first on November 9, the first day of the early signing period for college basketball. Graves and her mother sent the paperwork to the University of Tennessee after the ceremony at Clarksville High School in Clarksville, Tennessee. "I was overwhelmed," Graves said of the moment she put pen to paper. "It was exciting. It was surreal actually."

Jones followed suit the next day, November 10. "I worked this hard and got this far. I wasn't going to change my decision." Jones signed her letter of intent at Bob Jones High School in Madison, Alabama. Several thoughts can go through a parent's mind at that moment—thoughts of pride, accomplishment, and the passage of time—but LaTrish Jones had a basic one: "To be honest what was going through my mind was, 'Please don't sign on the wrong line,'" Jones said. The ceremony was not for show with replacement paperwork. The forms in front of Jasmine Jones were the originals and had to be faxed to Tennessee afterwards. "This was her original signature," LaTrish Jones said. "That is why I was a little nervous hoping that she did sign on the right line."

Carter inked her name on November 12, which coincided with her birthday. Her family and friends attended a celebration at Buford High School in Georgia, including some relatives who surprised her by making the drive from Ohio. "My family was there and my close friends. I will never forget it," Carter said. The Lady Vol coaches will also never forget the trio saying yes to Tennessee. Before they enrolled, the three shared what it meant to be a Lady Vol. "I literally cried when I received my first letter from the University of Tennessee in the eighth grade," Jones said. "I still have the letter. I had been a fan for as long as I can remember. It's hard to say where it all began, because one day I was a Moody Munchkin going to Alabama basketball, volleyball, gymnastics, soccer, and softball games and laughing and playing with huge Alabama football players, to all of a sudden being a Lady Vols fan. Other than Coach (Rick) Moody, Coach Summitt was the only other women's basketball coach that I knew of as a child.

"From my experiences in high school, I knew that I needed to really love my coach as well as the team that I would be playing with. I was really close with the coaches from Vanderbilt and Auburn, but I guess deep down Tennessee is where I belonged. My reaction to every other school's offer was calm and appreciative, but when I heard that UT wanted to offer, I screamed at the top of my lungs and scared everyone in the room. My mom told me to calm down and at least put some thought into it and not rush out of respect for the other schools and coaches. I committed after the UT vs. Vanderbilt game in Nashville on February 13, 2011. I needed to see both teams together so I could imagine my place on either team. I found myself secretly cheering for UT. Immediately after the game, I said that I am GOING to Tennessee and I called Coach Lockwood and Coach Summitt.

"I was very sad when I heard about Coach Summitt's diagnosis. I feel for Coach Summitt and her family, but I know that she is a strong woman and she caught the disease early enough for effective treatment. I chose to stay committed because she believed in me enough to make my dream a reality, so I refused to let her down or turn my back on her. The day that we found out the first thing that my mom spoke to me about was 'loyalty' and then she went on to ask me my thoughts and feelings on my decision and that she would support whatever I decide. I knew where I wanted to be, period.

"Pat believed in me enough to bring me into her program so I could only remain committed and true to my word. She entrusted me to represent the greatest college women's basketball program in history. She made my dream a reality and I refused to turn my back on her. It is hard to say how I feel about being the last class signed by Coach Summitt. It is a sad thing. I am honored, but I never wanted to be in her last class. I wanted to be able to tell future classes stories about her and joke around like players normally do. It is sad, but I am more dedicated to make her proud of her decision and belief in me."

Graves was equally as eloquent when asked to explain what it meant to her to join the long orange line. "The day I verbally committed, I went back and forth in my head asking, was it the right time; it was a huge decision, was I ready. I finally realized that I couldn't see myself anywhere else. It had gone beyond just the staff that I had seen over the years, the players, the crowds at the games or the championship trophies. It just felt like, 'This is where I belong.' When Coach Pat came out about her diagnosis, I didn't think about what that meant at first for me. I wanted to make sure that she was going to be all right. My decision to stay with my commitment had a little to do with all of the things I've mentioned before, but most of all I didn't see myself anywhere else. Even with the news of Coach Pat's retirement, my mind was not changed. I figured it would happen soon and understood that it was what was best for her and her health, which comes first. I get questioned all the time about how I feel about her retirement and my answer remains the same. I am a Lady Vol."

The three recruits formed a pact to stay, which pleased Carter to no end. "When Coach Summitt told me about her diagnosis, I didn't question my commitment at all," Carter said. "My dad told me, 'If you think twice about this then you need to reconsider where you want to go. You either bleed orange and white or you don't,' and I knew for a fact that I was sure I wanted to be a Lady Vol. When I tore my ACL, the Tennessee coaches all stuck with me and had faith in me. So when I heard about the early onset dementia diagnosis I knew I wanted to have faith in them.

"I come from a very religious family and I truly believe that Knoxville is where God wants me to be. I have always been at peace with my decision, even when Coach Summitt announced her disease and when she chose to step down as head coach. I have always wanted to be a Lady Vol, and that hasn't changed once. I knew for a fact that the announcement by Coach Summitt didn't affect my decision to be part of Tennessee women's basketball, but I remember wondering what Jasmine and Bashaara were going to do the day we all found out. It was a tweet from Shar and a text from Jasmine that let me know they were sticking with the Lady Vols just as much as I was. It was a relief to know that they felt as strongly about the program as I did and that we were going to all go together. It is an honor to be a part of the last class ever recruited and signed by Coach Summitt."

Warlick and Lockwood hit the road a day after the press conference. The staff's attention had to turn to recruiting with specific targets in the class of 2013. "We've held on to some great kids," Warlick said at the press conference. "I think the uncertainty about what was happening was a little bit of a concern, but immediately yesterday Dean and I got on the phone, and we've had nothing but positive reaction for myself and Dean staying and especially Pat staying on as well. It's been really a positive response for us on the recruiting side." It was also business as usual for Warlick and Lockwood as soon as the media responsibilities ended that Thursday. They were still permitted to have after-season workouts with the team in small groups—that window would close in a few days by NCAA rules—and were getting ready to head to Pratt Pavilion. Warlick still had Summitt's whistle around her neck while she went from camera to camera and reporter to reporter for the one-on-one interviews after the press conference ended. "I left at 5:30 the next morning and got on the UT plane and went to recruit," Warlick said. "I hit the ground running."

Warlick doesn't use the whistle at practice. Instead, it hangs behind her desk draped around the neck of a Summitt bobblehead doll on a bookshelf. When Warlick hit the recruiting trail, she fielded two remarks from other coaches at every stop. "People came up and said, 'Congratulations, I'm glad you got the job,' and 'How is Pat doing?'" Warlick said. Over the summer she moved from her smaller office to the one that had been occupied by Summitt. The office is spacious with a large-screen TV, whiteboard, conference table, couches, large desk, and bookshelves. The walls contain the presence of Summitt from photos with Warlick—including the whistle exchange—to magazines on the coffee table with Summitt on the cover. "It was hard for me to move in here," Warlick said. "It was Pat's office. I would have just stayed in my office over there where I was, but I needed to move. I always put things in perspective that I am carrying on a tradition for Pat as well as the university."

After that April press conference ended, all of the coaches and staff ended up in the basketball offices. Meshia Thomas, who had escorted Summitt to and from the media event, was nearby as always. Summitt had called Thomas the day before and asked her to be at the press conference. Thomas waited in the parking area next to the arena and escorted Summitt inside. "She said, 'Well, that's it.' It was a fog at that point," said Thomas, who stayed behind the black curtains during the press conference.

Summitt had been notified a week earlier by the White House that President Obama wanted to present her with the Presidential Medal of Freedom, the country's highest civilian honor. The ceremony was held in

Washington, D.C., on May 29, 2012. On April 19, 2012, the same day the White House announced the award, Summitt was in her office talking about it with what was now her former staff. A still shell-shocked Thomas waited outside the office door so that she could walk Summitt back to the car.

"Coach says, 'Well, let me call the president. Get the president on the phone.' At that point, the fog lifts," Thomas said. "I am thinking, 'Did she just say get the president on the phone?' Who says that? Who says: 'Get the president on the phone?'" A call was placed to the White House. "She said, 'I would like to speak to President Obama.' She's talking on the phone, OK, OK. She hangs up and says, 'They're going to call me back.' My mind is racing. I am thinking, 'Drones are overhead now. They're beaming down at us. They see me. They're trying to figure out who the heck just called us.' The phone rang again a few minutes later, and it was somebody from the White House. They left the message that he was in a meeting, but he would call her back. Coach looked at me and said, 'Hey, you want to go to the house? We're going to throw some steaks on the grill and wait for the president to call.' I was still like, 'Seriously? You're going to throw some steaks on the grill and wait for the president to call?'" Thomas had to get back to the campus police department, and Summitt told her to stop by her house after work and get a plate of food. For the record, President Obama called.

Summitt, of course, had gathered her staff in the basketball office conference room—the same place Lockwood later recalled that day with a shaking voice—before the news was announced. Lockwood stood and listened. "I stood right there," Lockwood said, nodding to a nearby wall. "I felt my eyes water up but afterwards I went in my office . . . and that is when it hit me. She just basically said, 'I've decided to step down. I think it's time. For my health and also the good of the program and moving forward. I think it's time for me to step aside.' That was it. It was vintage Pat in terms of pure, honest, basic. No fluff. It was direct and honest."

Summitt also told the players before the news became public. Taber Spani spent some time in Summitt's office for a one-on-one talk, a memory she will cherish forever. "I remember the day she officially retired, and we had an amazing talk in the office," Spani said. "It was just the two of us. I was so overwhelmed. I remember running out of the offices and running to my car and just breaking down. The fact that it was over and the fact that she had stepped down . . . my freshman and sophomore year I would have never, ever thought that's what would have happened. I think more than anything it hurt her because she just wanted to be there for everyone. She was so selfless like that."

During that time with Summitt, Spani saw not a head coach felled by Alzheimer's, but the strong woman who made so many youngsters like Spani pick up a basketball and want to play one day for Tennessee. "Definitely. 'This is Pat Summitt. This is who she is.' Obviously with the horrible disease of Alzheimer's she definitely had her good and bad days, but I do remember that meeting and I knew that who I was talking to was the same person who had been there for me when she was recruiting me and she wanted me to come to Tennessee," Spani said. "That was the same person who cared about me and my family and wanted to make sure her team would be OK."

The 2012 spring semester ended three weeks later, and the players scattered home before reporting back to campus in June to work as counselors at Tennessee's basketball camps. "I remember coming back for camp, going into my senior year, Holly had been named head coach, and Pat was head coach emeritus, and she said, 'Taber, I will be there for you. I am not going to leave. I will still be around,'" Spani said. "I get emotional now thinking about it. Those last players she was coaching, she wanted us to know that she cared. For someone who had accomplished so much and could retire, you could see her just wanting to reach out to her players. That is what I remember. That is what I think of when I think of Pat Summitt. I think of her character more than any plays she ever called or games she won or championships or banners hanging up of her. I think of who she was as a person."

37

PAT XO

Pat Summitt tributes became a crowded market after the iconic sports figure announced she had early onset dementia, coached a final season, stepped down with 1,098 wins, and then started a foundation with Tyler to combat Alzheimer's disease.

The honors for Summitt, including induction into the FIBA Hall of Fame in Switzerland, didn't slow down. ESPN entered the tribute market with a documentary of Summitt as part of the Nine for IX series—movies directed by women that focus on women's athletics. The challenge for film directors Lisa Lax and Nancy Stern Winters was to somehow find a fresh perspective. So Lax and Winters compiled a list of people who knew Summitt best, from players to coaches to friends, and sent small cameras with the instructions to turn the cameras on themselves and talk about Summitt.

The result was "Pat XO," a title that referred to standard coaching notations of Xs and Os when drawing up plays and also referred to a kiss and a hug. When the cameras came back full of stories with laughter and tears, it was apparent the double meaning would work well. "If this film had been done in a conventional way, I don't know that it would feel as revealing, as personal, as fresh as it does," said John Dahl, ESPN's executive producer for the series. "Lisa and Nancy make it work in a way that the mood varies. You get laughter. You get tears." It was a risky approach for filmmakers, because they essentially surrendered control of the camera. But what came back was a treasure trove of material with anecdotes from such well-known stars as pro quarterback and former Vol Peyton Manning and country music singer Kenny Chesney, a native of nearby Luttrell, Tennessee. The new challenge for the filmmakers was to somehow edit the submissions into a documentary that would run just under an hour.

The film debuted on June 26, 2013, at the Regal Riviera Stadium 8 in downtown Knoxville, an advance screening before the national ESPN release on July 9. Summitt and Pat Summitt Foundation co-founder Danielle Donehew attended, along with various athletics department administrators and university dignitaries. The media had a roped-off area, and orange carpet guided those on the invitation list into the theater. "On behalf of the Foundation, we are so thankful for ESPN and for Regal to step up and support Pat in this way and to help tell her story," Donehew told the assembled media. "I think it's told in a beautiful way from a lot of different perspectives."

Among those in attendance was North Carolina women's basketball coach Sylvia Hatchell, who left 600 summer campers in Chapel Hill and was flying right back afterwards. With minutes to spare before the movie started, she arrived via private plane and landed at a small airport just across the Tennessee River from downtown Knoxville. "I wanted to come see this," Hatchell said. "Pat has done so much for me."

Those who appeared in the film included former players Tamika Catchings, Shelley Sexton Collier, Chamique Holdsclaw, Michelle Marciniak, and Candace Parker; current Tennessee Coach Holly Warlick and Assistant Coach Dean Lockwood; Summitt's USA coach, Billie Moore; author Sally Jenkins, who has written three books with Summitt; former coach and now TV commentator Nell Fortner, who did a spot-on impression of Summitt; and Summitt's college teammate at Tennessee-Martin, Esther Hubbard, who nearly stole the show.

Parker and Summitt talked about Parker being held out of the first half of her homecoming game in Chicago in 2008 because she missed curfew on New Year's Eve. In turn, Marciniak, her parents, and longtime assistant Mickie DeMoss retold an oft-told story—and somehow made it even funnier—about how Summitt went into labor with her son-to-be on the recruiting visit to Macungie, Pennsylvania. Marciniak's mother told the coaches they could all just chat later. Tyler Summitt narrated the film, which is interspersed with videos, game footage, still photos, and his mother's words and memories. Less than seven months after the film's debut, Parker was courtside in Knoxville during the 2013–14 season on January 2, 2014, when Tennessee retired her jersey and hoisted a banner to the arena's rafters to join those of Catchings, Holdsclaw, Daedra Charles, Bridgette Gordon, and Warlick.

It had been a whirlwind week for Parker to end the year of 2013 as she flew from Russia to China to spend Christmas with her husband, Shelden Williams (China was his overseas pro location that winter) and then on to Los Angeles, her home base since she plays for the WNBA Sparks in the summer. By January 2 she was in Knoxville for the ceremony to retire her jersey, likely one of the easiest decisions Tennessee ever made. Parker's résumé as a Lady Vol fills pages in her official biography, but the relevant material was already in the rafters: two banners commemorating the 2007 and 2008 national titles.

Parker called me after cleaning out her shed, a rather pedestrian activity for one of the best players on the planet. She and her husband had sold their house in California and bought a new one—a moving process that was completed while both were overseas—so she was busy sorting items, unpacking, and organizing the house during her brief stay stateside. Parker managed to slip away for a few days from her professional team in Russia, the Euroleague's UMMC Ekaterinburg club, but she departed the day after the jersey ceremony for Yekaterinburg to rejoin her teammates. "My life is always crazy, so when it's not crazy, it's kind of weird. When I don't have anything to do after basketball, my husband said there is no way I will be able to just chill."

Williams wasn't able to make the trip to Tennessee, but Lailaa was present—and signed autographs at the tender age of 4—along with her mother, grandmother, and a host of other family members. Lailaa's father played for Duke, but Parker has made sure their daughter is all orange. "I don't think she understands (the jersey retirement), but she knows that we're going home to Knoxville and mommy played there, and she knows about mommy's coach and seeing her, so she is excited." Summitt and Warlick both accompanied Parker to center court for the ceremony, a gesture that meant so much to Parker. "I remember how players would come back and talk about how much Pat has impacted their everyday lives and the things that they do. And I don't think there are many people who have impacted my life like Coach. I think about her a lot when I am making decisions, when

I am going through different things. The things that she taught me when I was going to Tennessee help me and guide me into making decisions. She is an amazing and strong woman, so to have her there? It means a lot."

Lockwood has also remained close to Parker. They spent a lot of time together in Knoxville because she was constantly calling Lockwood to meet in the gym for extra shooting sessions. "I can't tell you how many times she blew my phone up, on a Saturday, on a Sunday, we weren't practicing or it was a (short) practice and she would come in early," Lockwood said. "I loved every minute of it. Here is a kid who loved working on her game. I don't think people really appreciated that about her. I think they looked at the talent she had and thought, 'Oh, she's so talented.'" Parker became the sixth Lady Vol player to have her jersey retired. Her No. 3 banner joined those of Warlick (No. 22), Holdsclaw (No. 23), Catchings (No. 24), Gordon (No. 30), and Charles (No. 32). Summitt also has a banner to commemorate her 38-year coaching career at Tennessee.

Parker played her last game for Tennessee on April 8, 2008, a 64–48 shutdown of Stanford that gave Summitt her eighth national title. She was the first pick in the WNBA draft the next day and won MVP and Rookie of the Year honors. While no official announcement was made until five years later on March 2, 2013, Parker's No. 3 wasn't given to any incoming player after she graduated. If a player asked, the answer was that No. 3 wasn't available. There was no doubt Parker's jersey belonged in the rafters of Thompson-Boling Arena.

When asked for a favorite Parker story, Lockwood mentioned the 2005–06 season, her first in orange after a redshirt year to heal from knee surgery. It is a story he tells when talking to players and coaches about the differences encountered when coaching women instead of men. "About eight or nine games into the season, she was shooting 56 to 57 percent," Lockwood said. "The coaching staff met every day to talk about practice. We have the team stat sheet out, and we're talking about what we need more of, how we're performing. One of the things Pat said right away is we have to get Candace Parker more shots. There wasn't a dissenting voice in the room. We were all like, 'Absolutely.' She was averaging about 15 points a game and doing it on about 10 or 11 shots. Pretty dang productive."

The seniors on the team were guard Shanna Zolman and center Tye'sha Fluker, so Summitt knew she would have to convince the redshirt freshman to take over a veteran club. Lockwood, who had coached men for decades before joining the Lady Vols, didn't realize that yet. Since Lockwood worked with the posts, he was assigned to deliver the order to Parker–shoot more.

"Pat said, 'Dean, I want you to bring her in to watch tape and approach her about this and then I will follow up with it. I am going to really drive it home, but I would like you to approach it with her,'" Lockwood said.

Parker was an avid viewer of game film, so Lockwood called her in to chat. "She was a visual person," he said. "She likes to see things. We're sitting there, and I said, 'Candace, I am going to show you something related to you, and what we are going to need from you going forward. I want you to look at the stat sheet, your stats in particular.' She was looking and looking and I said, 'Now, we're going to need something more from you. What do you think that is?' She kind of had a slight grin. She has a pretty high basketball IQ and she said, 'You want me to probably take more shots.' I said, 'You're dang right we do!'"

Parker was only a few games into her college career, but chatter had already started about national player of the year honors. She arrived as one of the most decorated high school players in Tennessee history. The fact she should be taking the most shots would be a given on a men's team. "The first thing out of her mouth was, 'I know Dean, but it's Shanna and Tye's team, and I want them to be OK with it.'" Lockwood was apoplectic. "We are talking about somebody who is in the conversation for player of the year," he said. "I said, 'I think everybody is going to be happy if we're winning games.' That is the one of the things I will always remember. Now, if you tell a guy you want more shots, he will step out of that door, and he's in the gym jacking shots. Candace was so team-oriented. That was just Candace."

Parker laughs now when Lockwood's story is relayed to her, but she offers a serious answer. "I think my family definitely keeps me humble," Parker said. "Anything I did as a kid, it was striving to do more and striving to be better. In Coach's words, I never arrived. I think that helped me be the best I can be. Obviously, basketball is a team sport and especially in women's athletics, emotions take a lot in the sport. From that aspect I want to make sure everybody is in a good place. Because when everybody is in a good place, it means that it's going to be a good season. You don't all have to like each other, but you have to be OK with decisions." Parker added, "I was young and I was a rookie, and I am a people pleaser."

Parker got more demonstrative later in her career. Summitt ran drills in which players sprinted up and down the court for at least three minutes and had to make left-handed layups on both ends. If anyone missed or used the right hand, the clock reset until the entire team completed the drill with no misfires. Parker never missed, but her teammates did. One day after repeated misses and restarts—the drill was exhausting because it was full court, game speed, and came at the end of practice—Parker exclaimed, 'Come on, it's a left-handed layup!'" Parker was a gifted player, but she made left-handed layups because she practiced them. "Early on people didn't appreciate how hard she worked on her game," Lockwood said. "Pratt Pavilion was one of the best things to happen to Candace Parker."

And Candace Parker was one of the best things to ever happen to Lady Vol basketball. The program paid its dues by preserving her jersey number in perpetuity. "What I am the most excited about—and this is going to sound crazy—but I can remember senior day and running out on the floor and being like, 'This is going to be the last time in Knoxville,'" Parker said days before the ceremony. "So to get this opportunity again and to be able to do it in front of people I love—my whole family is going to be there—I think it's special from that aspect. Knoxville is very special to me, and Tennessee means a great deal to me."

Parker was elated with the honor, but the loss of Summitt from the sidelines also struck her when she walked into the arena. "When I was there for my jersey retirement, it hits you. It's not going to be the same. You're sad that it's over. Pat always said, 'All good things come to an end. It happens. It's the way of life.' But it doesn't make it any less sad. A very big point in Tennessee history comes to an end. I honestly admire Holly a lot because I don't know many people who can take over and I don't know of anyone else I would want to take over the program because you need to keep it in familiar hands."

When "Pat XO" made its national debut, Glory Johnson, who was shown hugging Summitt in the locker room in Des Moines, was in the midst of her second WNBA season with the Tulsa Shock. (The franchise would relocate to Dallas in 2016.) The Shock had a road game in San Antonio, and Johnson recalled walking through the mall and then finding a place to eat. The television in the restaurant was tuned to ESPN, and the Nine for IX episode was airing. Johnson focused on the television and then fell apart. "I just started breaking down," Johnson said. "I was eating with people, and it was really awkward. Tears were falling. I couldn't stop them. I was with my friends and we were watching it, and I just starting crying. It's tough. It's really tough. Pat was like a mother to me." Johnson's professional basketball career keeps her busy nearly year-round, as she also plays overseas. But when she returned to her hometown, she found time to see Summitt.

Like Parker, Johnson slipped into Summitt's office as many times as she could, especially her senior year. Summitt handled one-on-one conversations very well in her final season. "Anytime I got a little free time I would go sit in Pat's office," Johnson said. "We would just sit down and talk for an hour. The more people that were brought into the situation or if there were more people in the room, I couldn't really talk to her like I used to. But whenever I was with her by myself, it was no problem. She was used to it, comfortable talking to me one-on-one in her office. Once there were a lot of people around, it was a harder situation. A lot of people don't understand that. It took a toll on Holly. It took a toll on the players not being able to talk to her when we needed to. We tried everything to get through it."

Vicki Baugh and Parker played one season together and remain close friends, and both were also extremely close to Summitt. Baugh called Parker that final season just to talk. "All of the lessons Pat taught us prepared us for this," Parker said. "She would always tell us, 'Things aren't fair. You don't have a choice in the hand you're dealt, but you have a choice in the way you deal with the hand you're dealt.' I think that team dealt with it the way Pat would, the way Pat did. That is what is so special about it. I was proud of them. I was really proud of them. I know they had goals of going all the way and going to the Final Four but just for what they overcame, I was really proud of them."

At the end of the "XO" film, Pat Summitt is in tears when she discusses her retirement. "I didn't want to, but I felt like I needed to step down," she said, words met with tears from many of the attendees at the exclusive Knoxville screening. As the film ended, Summitt received a standing ovation and hugs from well-wishers as they departed the theater.

That the film would resonate so well in Knoxville wasn't a surprise; it also made an impact upon national release. "I think throughout women's basketball people are going to see why Pat Summitt won nearly 1,100 games," Dahl said. "It's not just about Xs and Os. It's about how to connect with her players, with her assistant coaches, her values, what she stands for. If you watch this film, you'll understand why she's achieved what she's achieved in life."

Lockwood breaks down in the film when he talks about Summitt, her disease, and her legacy in basketball, and Parker wasn't surprised to see her former post coach get so emotional. "Dean is a passionate guy. He is extremely passionate," Parker said. "He truly believes in everything that Pat has said. He truly believes in her words and her work ethic. It was really hard for me to watch that. It hits you."

38

PAT SUMMITT'S FINAL CHAMPIONSHIP

As the confetti fell to the court in Tampa , Florida, after a national title game played before 21,655 fans, the majority of whom were wearing orange, no one present, including me, would have ever thought it would be Pat Summitt's final NCAA championship. "No, not at all," a wistful Candace Parker said. "Obviously, I didn't think that would be her last title."

The Lady Vols dismantled Stanford by a score of 64–48 and became the first team in women's college basketball history to twice win back-to-back national championships.

When Pat Summitt climbed the ladder April 8, 2008, to snip the final pieces of net, the roar seemed as loud as when the final seconds ticked off the clock and the players rocked in each other's arms. Tennessee finished

---

Author's note: Tennessee got to the title game in 2008 because of the brilliance and relentless preparation of Summitt. That Final Four is worth its own chapter.

36–2 and completed a Final Four in which it held both opponents to under 50 points. The Lady Vols defeated LSU 47–46 on a Sunday to make it to the title game that Tuesday against Stanford, 35–5. "We loved the fact that nobody picked us to win," senior guard Alexis Hornbuckle said. "That was what motivated us truly. We were reading an article where it said Tennessee is not going to be able to hold Stanford to under 50 points because they're basically offensive machines. We held them to 48."

Debby Jennings and Dean Lockwood had a direct hand in getting the Lady Vols so motivated for the title game. Jennings, affectionately called "DJ" by all teams for years, had gathered and printed the predictions of national writers. Senior center Nicky Anosike read the remarks out loud to the team in the locker room at what was then called the St. Pete Times Forum. "DJ had six prognosticators, and they had their predictions and why, and five of the six had picked Stanford," Lockwood said. "Nicky read excerpts of some of the stuff they said and then we taped it on the head of this mannequin." The players were worked into a fervor with shouts of "that doesn't matter to us, we know who we are," Lockwood said.

Then, Lockwood grabbed the baseball bat and swung. The head exploded, and the mannequin was instantly dismembered. "That was the coup de grace," Lockwood said. "I hit it in the head and it was like special effects. The head just popped. It was a direct hit and it was boom! It couldn't have been better if I planned it." The players charged out of the locker room with a last-minute directive from the coaching staff to "put some major defense on them and let's go bring it." "I sensed that this team was ready to step up and defend Stanford in a way that we could be disruptive and be successful," Pat Summitt said the morning after the title game in a classic understatement.

It certainly wasn't an easy path to be able to hoist that trophy, but no national title ever is. Even the explosive and undefeated 1998 team had to overcome a 12-point deficit with seven minutes to play against North Carolina to reach the Final Four in Kansas City. The Elite Eight game was played in Memorial Gym in Nashville, with its odd configurations of benches on the baseline and no basketball stanchion. Instead, the backboard was held in place by an arch-like structure with two poles anchored on either side. One pole was very close to the bench, and Summitt, with arms folded, was leaning on the pole, intently watching the action.

Her parents and siblings were seated directly behind Tennessee's bench, and the game became memorable not just for the comeback, but also because Summitt's sister, Linda Atteberry, yelled at her to stop leaning on the pole and start coaching because she had nonrefundable plane tickets for the entire family to Kansas City. Tennessee won its sixth national title a week later by pasting Arkansas and Louisiana Tech. Title number seven came in Cleveland, Ohio, in 2007 and required Tennessee to beat Pittsburgh on its home floor in the second round and then head to Dayton, which had been called the Region of Death with Tennessee, Oklahoma, defending champion Maryland, and Ohio State all on one side of the bracket. But Marist College and Ole Miss had dispatched some giants along the way and arrived in Dayton with Tennessee and Oklahoma. The Lady Vols eliminated Marist and then Ole Miss forced an up-tempo attack against the Sooners, who wilted in the heat.

A week before the Dayton Regional, the area had been hit with a snowstorm. But teams and fans were greeted with outside temperatures of 80 degrees and the odd sight of large piles of shoveled snow in the parking lot. Dayton Arena wasn't air-conditioned. The football locker room had been converted into the media working room, and as temperatures rose, so did the stench of stale odors. Large fans were set up and doors opened, where possible, but writers on deadline were sweating—literally. Media row courtside was even worse, as there wasn't any airflow. Anyone in a suit jacket or long sleeves—standard basketball attire for the NCAA tourney—was drenched in sweat. Courtside temperatures measured at over 90 degrees. The mother of Lady Vol forward Sidney Spencer went to a local retail store to buy shorts and T-shirts so she could sit somewhat comfortably in the stands.

The Lady Vols had spent the week practicing at Stokely Athletics Center, which has since been torn down, because Thompson-Boling Arena was in use for another function. Stokely was a hot box and it had been warm in Knoxville, so the Lady Vols had no issues with the Dayton heat. Ole Miss had trapped Oklahoma relentlessly with double teams to force turnovers, but Tennessee, led by Parker, just passed over them to open teammates and smothered Ole Miss with a score of 98–62. A week later Tennessee was back in Ohio and defeated North Carolina in the semifinal, again wiping out a 12-point deficit, this time with eight minutes to play. They did not allow one Tar Heel field goal during that stretch, and afterward they dispatched Rutgers for title number seven.

Summitt's eighth national title didn't come easy, either. The Lady Vols escaped the Oklahoma City Regional with an Elite Eight win over Texas A&M. The Aggies could do nothing with Parker—she was on pace for 40 points—but then her left shoulder dislocated as she stole a pass in the first half. She kept her dribble down the sideline with her right hand while her left arm swung like sea oats in the wind, and when one Texas A&M player attempted to steal the ball, she recoiled in horror at the sight. Parker came back in the second half with a brace but was clearly hindered. She had tallied 16 points in the first half and managed 10 in the second in a physical contest.

Tennessee trailed 42–37 in the second half with both teams clamping down on defense, but Parker put Tennessee ahead with two free throws, 43–42, with less than four minutes to play. Parker lost the ball in the lane late in the game but managed to tip it to Hornbuckle, who was deep on the perimeter. Hornbuckle tallied her points with defense, stick-backs, and athletic forays to the rim, but she drained an NBA-range three-pointer with the shot clock nearly at zero for a 48–43 lead with 48.8 seconds left that seemed to finally deflate the Aggies. The Lady Vols sealed the 53–45 win for another Final Four berth.

Texas A&M Coach Gary Blair was gracious—and funny—in defeat. He got his own national title three years later in 2011 after defeating Notre Dame, the school the Lady Vols beat in Oklahoma City in the Sweet 16 before facing A&M in that 2008 Elite Eight. "Neither team can look back at one particular play that just made it, because even if Hornbuckle would have missed that shot from 40 feet, Batman could have come in and got the rebound and dunked on us," Blair said, referring to Parker, who dunked seven times in her college career, none more memorable than the one she threw down in 2007 on Connecticut in Hartford during a national CBS broadcast.

The Lady Vols arrived in Tampa with an ailing Parker, who was determined to play. She was the consensus No. 1 draft pick—the Los Angeles Sparks drafted her first the day after the national title game—and wanted to end her Tennessee career with another national title. But LSU awaited in the semifinal with the 6'6" Sylvia Fowles at center, and the battles between the Lady Vols and the Lady Tigers had been epic. LSU defeated Tennessee in Knoxville that season, costing the Lady Vols the SEC regular season title, while the Lady Vols claimed the SEC Tournament title in Nashville with a win over LSU.

Parker's shoulder had dislocated again in Tampa while brushing her teeth. She had instructed Vicki Baugh to get Moshak, and instead of calling her as Parker intended, Baugh ran down the hotel hallway yelling for Moshak. Parker was in pain—a national ESPN commentator said LSU should hit Parker in the shoulder until it brought tears to her eyes, which outraged Tennessee fans—but the Lady Vols prevailed, 47–46, when Hornbuckle rebounded an Anosike miss with 1.7 seconds left in the game. Hornbuckle, who had been 0–7 to that point, grabbed the ball and shot in one motion. When the ball settled through the net, a mere .7 seconds remained in the game.

The ever-prepared Summitt had used a segment of practice before the 2008 Final Four to address this precise situation. She put an uncanny seven seconds on the clock and set the parameters for the players. They had to go the length of the floor to win the game. Parker was to bring the ball down court and either go to the rim or pass to an open teammate. Everyone else crashed the boards. They ran the drill several times, sometimes with seven seconds left, sometimes with eight or five seconds. They practiced the drill after a made free throw, missed free throw, and off an in-bounds pass.

Just two weeks later on the game's biggest stage, LSU's Erica White made two free throws to give the Lady Tigers a one-point lead, 46–45, with 7.1 seconds to go. LSU called timeout to set its defense. Tennessee used the timeout to go over what it had recently practiced back home in Knoxville. Parker wore a long-sleeve shirt under her uniform to cover the shoulder and try not to call attention to the brace, though she was ailing and enduring a miserable offensive night, shooting 6–27 from the field. But Assistant Coach Nikki Caldwell had no doubt whose hands she wanted the ball in at crunch time. Parker had run the play to perfection in practice. She had gone to the basket at times or passed off to a cutting teammate. "We have a coaching staff that has prepared us for every situation. In practice we did that play over and over and over again," Parker said. "Different ways with different people in different positions. I think at the time some of us didn't quite understand coach's thoughts and why we were doing it over and over again."

"They're still second-guessing me," Summitt said to much laughter during the press conference the day after the national title game for the winning team. "It's weird how everything seems to at the end just come together," Parker said. "What was so special about our team is even with seven seconds left and down by one point, we were going to find a way to win. That's what great teams do. Some people call it luck, but I call it pulling together and winning the game. The last seven seconds of the game encompassed everything that we are the whole entire season." Parker got the in-bounds pass from Hornbuckle, who took off down court as if shot out of a cannon. She trailed the play in case Parker got trapped, but Parker had run the drill against quick and agile male practice players. The LSU defense, by comparison, offered little resistance. Parker was at Tennessee's end in just under four seconds, and as the LSU post players collapsed on her, Parker fired a pass to Anosike, who shot and missed with 2.5 seconds to go.

But Hornbuckle grabbed the ball and shot in one motion with 1.7 seconds showing on the clock. She banked in the offensive rebound, and .7 seconds were left as the ball settled through the net. "It felt like a lifetime," Hornbuckle said. "We knew seven seconds was a long time, especially when you break it down to some of the sprints that we do, and we drill it in practice. When it came down to it we listened to what she wanted us to do, and we executed it. Luckily we crashed the boards, and Candace had very good court vision to drop the pass to Nicky Anosike."

"And I blew it," Anosike said.

"Luckily in the end everything fell together," Hornbuckle said, a modest statement considering how it came together for Tennessee.

"It's OK, Nick," Parker said.

"It's all right. You got a good follow-up by Alexis," Summitt said as the players smiled on the dais.

A month later Summitt was replaying the moment in her head. "The thing that it says about that team is that they didn't panic," Summitt said. "They had a lot of composure, and they found a way to win. Our timeout was very calm. As I told them, seven seconds is a long time. No one hit a panic button by any means." Summitt and Assistant Coach Dean Lockwood didn't see the final shot, which Hornbuckle put up from the left side of the basket. The Tennessee bench faced the right side of the basket, and Lockwood got screened off by an official.

Summitt's mind flashed to the Rutgers game and the ensuing clock controversy when Anosike was fouled with .2 seconds left and hit two free throws to win the game, so her eyes went to the shot clock instead of the basket. Summitt saw Anosike's miss and was wondering how much time would be left to try to get the ball back. Next thing she knew, Tennessee had points on the scoreboard. "I felt very fortunate," Summitt said. "It could have gone either way. It's unfortunate either team had to lose, but I was elated for our team. I couldn't see the shot. I had to see that on replay on tape because I was looking at the clock after the whole Rutgers thing."

Associate Head Coach Holly Warlick had moved into position on the bench to see the shot by Hornbuckle. "The official was right there," Lockwood said. "I didn't see it. I asked Holly, 'Who made the shot?' Lex? Lex! Incredible." The coaching staff was expecting LSU to try to deny Parker the ball or double her if she got it. But Parker cut to Hornbuckle at an angle to receive the entry pass and got up the floor in just a few dribbles. "We were surprised we were able to get it in to her," Lockwood said. "There is a lot of time, but there's not a lot of time to fool around. You've got to go right to the basket. We knew it was going to be a straight drive or a kick. Fortunately, Lex was there. We were confident in our team. In your mind you're staring the reality in the face that this could be it. I really thought we were going to get a shot, but sometimes it goes and sometimes it doesn't."

Preparation came into play on the second shot, too. Summitt was adamant during the practice drills that everyone go to the glass in those waning seconds. There was no need to stay back on defense, not with the clock about to hit zero. On one occasion during one of the drill repetitions, Summitt noticed that all five players on the floor didn't hit the boards. She blew the whistle and lined them up for a wicked series of wind sprints. "I remember," Summitt said. "We're going to stand around and watch and, yeah, I put them on the baseline." LSU had no chance at a defensive board, which would have won the game and ended the Lady Tigers' futility in the Final Four. LSU had made five consecutive Final Fours to that point and lost every time in a semifinal game.

Hornbuckle and Angie Bjorklund had the left side of the basket blocked. Anosike was still under the basket, and Parker had scooted around to the opposite side from where she made the pass. Shannon Bobbitt was staying with White on the perimeter. "That was habit and preparation more than luck," Lockwood said of the ending. Hornbuckle had a heads-up play to set up the final seven seconds, but had Tennessee not won the game, it would have been second-guessed until Lady Vol time eternal.

Hornbuckle had missed a shot with the shot clock expiring and White was headed down the sideline. Hornbuckle reached in and fouled White for two reasons: LSU was 5–17 from the free throw line to that point, and she didn't want the Lady Tigers to hit a go-ahead shot that left little to no time on the clock for Tennessee. White hit both free throws, and Hornbuckle got her redemption in the end. Both Lockwood and Summitt said it was the right decision by the senior guard to foul White. "In that situation you're going to get the ball back if they score, but your time is going to be very limited," Lockwood said. "At least give us an opportunity to have the ball with a shot to win the game."

Hornbuckle capped off the game by swiping LSU's in-bounds pass—she graduated from Tennessee with the school record of 373 steals—and the celebration began. Anosike, who had written a pact for the Lady Vols outlining how to repeat and vowed to live in a cardboard box if the Lady Vols lost in Tampa, embraced her fellow senior and repeatedly thanked her as the Lady Vol fans in the St. Pete Forum exploded. The Lady Vols finished their quest two nights later on April 8, 2008, with the takedown of Stanford, despite all the national doubt that any team could slow down the Cardinal offense. Coaches of all sports know defense trumps pretty offense every time.

The day after the national title game, Summitt and the five starters met with the media in an early-morning press conference in a ballroom at the downtown Hyatt in Tampa. The official trophy presentation had occurred after midnight in a ballroom in the same hotel, and the WNBA draft was only a few hours away. "Obviously, we haven't had a whole lot of sleep and certainly last night was a very special night," Summitt said in a voice that left no doubt both how tired and how happy they were. "These young ladies, they made it happen with leadership, the mindset, the defensive intensity and the execution overall. It was very important to our coaching staff and obviously to our seniors that this group go back-to-back with their national championships. They will always be very, very special to me, to the University of Tennessee and to all Lady Vols fans. I'm just excited for what lies ahead for them as they continue their basketball careers. They have definitely left their mark on the University of Tennessee and the basketball program."

None of the players knew it at the time, but they were the team that would claim Summitt's last national championship. "Given that it was, it means a lot to be a part of it," Parker said. "If it's possible to make that championship even more special, that definitely makes it that. That season was hard. It is hard to stay motivated after you win one. We had our ups and downs that season. We had our mother-daughter relationship. It's not the national championship that I'll remember; it will be the bus rides, the conversations, the flights, the timeouts, the things we had off the court that I will remember most about it. That's what stands out in my mind, and that's what is so special about it."

39
THE LEGACY

Dementia may have prematurely dimmed Pat Summitt's flame, but it will never be extinguished. It is carried by those who became coaches because of Summitt, by players who now know they can overcome any challenge in life, and by assistants like Dean Lockwood, who admired Summitt while on another staff and later joined the Lady Vols because of his profound respect for her.

"Her legacy is and will be a leader of character who brought out the very best in the people around her, who had a passion to bring out the best in people around her," Lockwood said. "She was a tremendous competitor and a champion, not only in terms of winning eight national championships, 1000-plus games, and the 100 percent graduation rate, but I think above and beyond that she wanted the people around her to be equipped and very well prepared for whatever life held for the challenges and the opportunities that were going to come. She was a leader of tremendous character, someone of incredible impact. You couldn't help but be around Pat and be impacted positively.

"I was an assistant coach for five years down the hallway watching her practice, watching her interact, how she handled herself. Working with her for eight years took it to another level. I can only imagine playing for her and that experience. Her legacy will be as a leader of tremendous impact who cared for her people, wasn't afraid to hold people accountable, challenge them, and be demanding, but at the same time love them. I think that's rare that you can do all of those things in good measure and do them well. That's what Pat did."

Summitt never sought the accolades. She always said she wanted her coaching tenure to be remembered because of what her players did, how they succeeded after leaving her program. Candace Parker, one of the greatest basketball players in the world, got emotional and then animated when talking about her coach. "A lot of people talk the talk, but while you're talking the talk, she's walking the walk. While everybody else is busy doing other stuff, Pat is working. And Pat's backing up what she says. And Pat's living what she speaks. I think that is what her legacy is. There is no stronger woman that I've ever known. That's what she'd want her legacy to be."

The final season was a salute to that legacy as fans roared upon seeing her and came to their feet, even on the road. "Every single place that we went, whether home or away, every game was a tribute to Pat," Glory Johnson said. "They had signs in the stands for Pat, and they were clearly fans of the other team. They were loyal, loyal basketball fans. I think everyone let her know and acknowledged that she had done so much for the game. Every time she walked out, it was a standing ovation from everybody. Everyone wanted her to know how much they appreciated her. Everyone did that, no matter where we played."

Lockwood and the other coaches couldn't help but notice the signs and hear the shouts of support. But they also had to get the players ready for tipoff, because when the clock started, the opposing team wanted a win as much as Tennessee did. The pleasantries were for before and after the game, not during it. "I burrowed in even more. I would take a second and appreciate it, but I burrowed in even more," Lockwood said, "I was so focused on we've got to help this team be ready, and we've got to help Pat. I was so appreciative to people for showing that to Pat, but this is going to be over and a ball is going up and there's a game going on. We had to make sure our players were focused and ready, and we've got to show that to our players. People waiting for her before our games, after our games, people coming up to us, 'Can you get her to sign this?' It felt like a farewell tour."

Mickie DeMoss had seen firsthand the effect Summitt had on attendance on the road and the reaction of fans, but that final season stood out even to a seasoned coach. "It was quite impressive," DeMoss said. "I don't think it affected the team in a negative way. I think, if anything, it inspired them. It was unbelievable in certain arenas. It was very touching and you stopped to think, wow, what an impact this woman has had on a lot of programs, not just Tennessee." Meighan Simmons agreed with that assessment. Each game felt like a shot to underscore the importance of Summitt to the game. "It did because of the impact that she has made on so many people before anybody knew about this illness. People respected her in a manner where you had to celebrate her some way, somehow," Simmons said. "I wasn't just playing for the University of Tennessee. You were playing for her. For the team, we took that as a way of motivation."

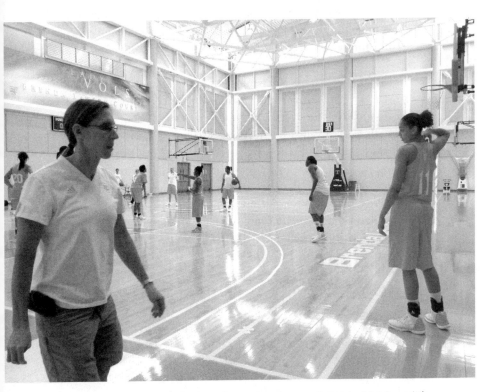

Jenny Moshak, left, was never far from the court and was a vital part of Pat Summitt's staff for years.

Responsible for the players' physical well-being, Jenny Moshak watched thousands of hours of basketball games and practices in a different way than anyone else. She watched to see how players moved, how they landed, how long they took to get up after a collision. She watched them in timeouts, especially during the final season when she knew the players were absorbing one of the biggest blows of a young person's life. She saw Summitt narrow her focus and stay engaged with players whose eyes always went to hers. "She did still have a presence. She could see the team take the information from Holly and then look to her," Moshak said. "Pat would shake her head, affirming. There were challenges to it, but there was amazing support. Every time she walked in the gym, the crowds, the applause. It wasn't officially a farewell tour, but it was in a sense a farewell tour, and you look back on it, it was a farewell tour, but that wasn't the plan going into the season.

"Everyone rallied around it. It made me proud to be associated with someone who had this much influence. We always knew she did, but you come into a situation like this and it's a whole other level of fame. She was now going to be the symbol for so many people. She put a name and a face to it, to step out there and continue to be the force for women, for women's basketball, for this disease, for the success of Tennessee. I think that said a lot." Moshak didn't have any issues communicating with Summitt that season. She knew sometimes information would need to be repeated and she did so in matter-of-fact fashion. "She would ask me a question about a player and then she would ask me again," Moshak said. "You just answer it again. It was very simple. That's all we needed to do. Treat her with respect."

Moshak was always a confidante for the players. They trusted her with every aspect of their health. She also was a sounding board for any of the typical college player issues—relationships, tough class, family matters. When the players gathered that summer day and heard Summitt tell them that she had early onset dementia, the words of Cierra Burdick and Alicia Manning stuck with Moshak because they were so forceful and supportive. "Everybody said something, but you remember the ones that speak out more. Cierra was very outspoken. A-Town was very outspoken. There were not a lot of questions asked, just a support atmosphere. Pat was very determined, and the team rallied around that. There were tears. A bit of shock. It wasn't about the basketball. It was about Pat. What I wanted to do was take the role of, 'how can I help in any way.' And several of the players did come to me later and just process about why, what does this mean, what is this going to look like, and how, in retrospect, some things made a little more sense. Some of the feelings they had from those instances mellowed."

Angie Bjorklund was one of the players who witnessed Summitt at one of her peaks—the national title of 2008—and was also on hand for the manifestation of behavioral changes, such as the forgetfulness and frustration on the part of the head coach that emerged during the 2010–11 season, Bjorklund's final one at Tennessee. Bjorklund had been in plenty of team meetings in her four-year career. She couldn't imagine one as devastating as hearing that Summitt had dementia just days before preseason workouts began. "When I heard I was in tears," Bjorklund said. "Fight for her and be motivated for her. But it would be a really tough situation."

The season took a toll on Holly Warlick. Not only did she have to become a de facto head coach, she was a daily witness to watching a woman she worshiped be affected by an insidious disease. "Looking back I don't know how I did. It is not a pity party. I don't know how I did it," Warlick said. "It was a just a tough year." Warlick hugged Summitt at basketball games, especially when the opposing team had former Lady Vols on the staff. Against Wichita State in the 2014–15 season, Warlick presented former Lady Vol Jody Adams, the Shockers' head coach, and Bridgette Gordon, an assistant, with flowers. The three then walked to Summitt's front row seat to hug their former head coach. Warlick went to see Summitt on a regular basis to visit and talk. Summitt settled into a routine and managed the illness as well as she could before her death in 2016, but Warlick remains crestfallen at what befell the iconic woman who deserved a better ending to her coaching career. "Every time you leave and get in the car, you cry on the way out. You just start crying," Warlick said of the visits to see Summitt at her home and then at the assisted living facility.

It was Summitt's sense of humor that was much needed that final season, from her joking about forgetting about bad losses to imitating her staff. "You can't help but laugh," Warlick said. "Laughter was huge for her. We had great times. One thing Pat created is we worked hard, but we played hard." Summitt was known to enjoy a glass or two of fine red wine. She also loved to play cards–and was quite adept at it. Summitt picked up card playing from her mother, Hazel Head. "She would go to New Orleans," Warlick said. "She loves to play blackjack. She is excellent at cards."

Summitt could still summon her thunder when needed during that last season—video clips taken inside the locker room by the Lady Vols, especially in the early NCAA rounds in Chicago, showed vintage delivery by the head coach. Warlick remembered times earlier in their assistant careers when she and Mickie DeMoss thought the team needed a break. "We would say, 'Pat, the kids look tired. Why don't we take off?' She would say, 'We can't take off! Especially on the weekend. They don't have class. We can practice longer.' She would say, 'Where do you two want to go? Y'all must want to go somewhere.' If we wanted one little day off, she would think Mickie and I had an ulterior motive." During the final season, Warlick suggested some down time for the players and got an entirely different reaction from Summitt. "I would say, 'I don't know if we should practice. They look tired.' And Pat would say, 'They need some rest. You need to give them some time off.' I was like, 'Oh, my God. It's total reversal of everything. Have times changed!'"

Warlick was Summitt's heir apparent. She held the team together after the devastating announcement about Summitt's disease. Most importantly, she and Dean Lockwood provided continuity to a program that had been led for nearly 40 years by the same woman. The parents of the class of 2012 recruits were at peace with their daughters sticking with their commitment to Tennessee because while the impact of Summitt's illness rumbled the earth beneath orange-and-white sneakers, Warlick and Lockwood remained to stabilize the program.

The final class of Andraya Carter, Bashaara Graves and Jasmine Jones epitomized Pat Summitt. They didn't start college with a lot of accolades, but they arrived ready to get to work. "All three are just wonderful kids," said LaTrish Jones, Jasmine's mother. "Bashaara is a workhorse. She just goes in and works. Draya is an unreal athlete and her basketball IQ is phenomenal. All three are outstanding. They look like her ballplayers. That kind of breaks my heart that they never got a chance to play for Pat." Summitt was in her first season as head coach emeritus when the trio arrived on campus. Cierra Burdick, Isabelle Harrison and Ariel Massengale were now sophomores. Summitt was a frequent visitor to practice during the trio's freshman year in college and that helped Carter adjust. "She will still comment on the game. She gives you advice. That is a blessing," Carter said.

It was reassuring to the parents that Warlick was there to greet their daughters, especially in the latter part of their career when Summitt's appearances were much less frequent. "Once we started doing the whole recruiting thing, her passion for Tennessee was always there," said Keinya Graves, Bashaara's mother. "Tennessee was the first one to really show interest in her. My main concern was who was going to be coaching. I know my child. She has a hard enough time adjusting. Dean and Holly had called and said, 'We are still going to be here.' I said, 'You know them.'" The announcement that it would be Warlick with Lockwood also staying brought as much relief to the Graves' household as it did to Carter's family. "I could not have pictured anybody else being the head coach," said Jessica Lhamon,

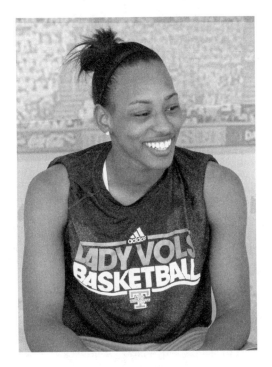

Bashaara Graves, shown as a freshman in Holly Warlick's first season, was a key piece of the 2012 recruiting class who stayed together after Pat Summitt's diagnosis.

Andraya's mother. "The program is the same. It is a loyalty, family thing, and that will never change. Andraya and Holly have a special bond, and it was an honor to be a parent of Holly's first team."

Carter's stepfather, Tyke Lhamon, wholeheartedly endorsed Warlick as the next head coach. She was in his living room with Summitt, and he knew Warlick would be the best choice going forward. "I wanted it to be somebody that was in the program, because that was going to keep the program the way it was," he said. "I thought if they brought somebody else in, they would have to put their stamp on it and change some things, which may not be for the better."

Tyke Lhamon also saw the softer side of Summitt when Carter's freshman season was cut short by shoulder surgery. She had dislocated her shoulder late in her senior year in high school, and it kept popping out during games at Tennessee, sending the first-year guard to the floor in agony. Even the act of reaching into the backseat for her book bag could loosen Carter's shoulder. Carter could still redshirt because she had only played a few games, so the decision was made to stop her freshman season and operate on the shoulder to stabilize and repair the joint. "When Pat found out, she actually cried," Tyke Lhamon said. "That went a long way with what kind of program it was. It wasn't all about fans and money. It was about the players."

Warlick was the perfect successor to Summitt. She played for the iconic coach, joined her on the sideline in 1985, and most importantly, embraced Summitt as head coach emeritus. Following Summitt is akin to replacing Bear Bryant or Dean Smith. Warlick, a native Knoxvillian and lifelong Tennessean—minus two coaching stops in Virginia and Nebraska during the 1980s—was devoted to Summitt, who would be around for practices and games as much as she chose to be before her death in 2016. Warlick welcomed Summitt's presence, whereas a new coach without extensive ties to Tennessee could have found it unnerving.

Summitt came to practice, put her arm around Warlick, and smiled. Warlick said her most important job was to take care of Summitt. "She would say, 'Well, Holly's the coach now.' And I would say, 'Oh, no. You're the boss.'" In Warlick's first season the Lady Vols reached the Elite Eight and lost to Louisville, 86–78. She remembered NCAA tourney defeats while coaching with Summitt, who seethed for months afterward. "When we would lose, we would go back and beat ourselves up to a point where we would get so exhausted, we would need to sleep for five days," Warlick said. "We were angry. Angry at the kids. Angry at ourselves. Watch the tape until you can't watch it anymore. I did that with the Louisville game. I called Pat. We didn't take care of the ball. We missed layups. We missed free throws. I should have done this. We should have done that. I am just ranting and raving. She just listened. There was dead silence on the phone. She said, 'Holly?' I said, 'Yeah?' She said, 'You've just got to let it go.' I was like, 'OK . . . Summitt, you're exactly right.'"

Warlick also had a legacy to maintain, and that started with recruiting. The score of that loss was eye-popping because 78 points should get a team to the Final Four. But it won't if the opposing team scores 86. Warlick decided to reshape Tennessee's defense to a retro look—a quintessential Summitt one of pressure and trapping. Warlick also had to sign a blockbuster class in 2013 to send a national signal that Tennessee was here to stay. She and Lockwood made a conscious decision to target key players in 2013—ones who could also defend—even if it meant getting behind in the classes of 2014 and 2015. The Lady Vols had to make a statement with the first signing class after Summitt exited.

Jannah Tucker, a top 10 recruit from Maryland, was the first to say yes to Warlick knowing that Summitt would not be on the sideline. She entered

Lady Vol lore in June 2013 when she made a verbal commitment to Tennessee. "It was a major statement," Warlick said. Tucker, whose college career was ultimately waylaid by knee injuries, was one of the three primary targets identified by Warlick and Lockwood. The other two were Jordan Reynolds and Mercedes Russell, both from Oregon. They came on board after official visits in October 2012 and signed scholarship papers the next month, along with Tucker. Lockwood and Warlick had plowed considerable resources into the three. "We had great relationships with all three of them," Warlick said.

Of course, Warlick and Lockwood had to combat negative recruiting throughout the process. Rival schools told recruits that Warlick would never win in the SEC—and then she took the league crown in her debut season. Warlick also had to prove that a top program could still recruit without ethical lapses, such as making staff hires primarily to sign the connected high school player, or outright cheating, a situation that has escalated in women's basketball. As salaries for head coaches climbed, the pressure to keep those lucrative jobs—and win—led to a willingness to break rules. The NCAA, as of now, hasn't intervened in any significant way. Warlick won't betray Summitt's trust. "We're not going to," Warlick said. "Everything that she said and built, it empowered me. This is the only way I know. I am not going to cheat. I am determined. I am thankful. I know her values. That is what has been taught to me."

Taber Spani played her senior year with Warlick as her head coach. Spani is a competitor with a warrior mentality similar to that of Summitt. She is also fiercely loyal, both to Summitt and to Warlick. "Before the season started I was trying to think of how I could honor Pat and yet honor Holly as well," Spani said. "I didn't want to take anything away from Holly, and she was my head coach. And yet Pat Summitt was also my head coach, and I just love her so much. In that first game, she sat right behind the bench, so she was right there and I could go and give her a hug. I just wanted to honor her. It was calming. It was an outward expression of me being able to cherish Pat."

Summitt's son, Tyler, was on track to be one of her greatest legacies to the game. He became a head coach at the age of twenty-three—one year older than his mother—when once-storied Louisiana Tech hired him to take over the Lady Techsters. In hindsight, he wasn't ready for such responsibility, and his downfall was as rapid as his ascent into the upper echelon of the coaching ranks.

Tyler Summitt had asked Mickie DeMoss to join him in Ruston, and she would end up becoming interim head coach of the program for a very brief period after he was forced to step down. DeMoss is a Louisiana native and graduate of Louisiana Tech. The request made sense, but DeMoss wasn't certain about getting back into the college game and the rigors of recruiting. She had planned to stay in the WNBA and was part of the staff, led by Tennessee native Lin Dunn, that seized the Indiana Fever's first WNBA title. "When he first mentioned something to me I was like, 'Huh?' And he said, 'I know you think I am probably crazy for asking you this.' I said, 'Yeah.' After a few days I called him back," DeMoss said.

DeMoss noted that she didn't want to be the recruiting coordinator—she had done that at Tennessee and it was an exhausting role—but that she would return to the sideline. "He said, 'I want you for a lot more than recruiting.' After we talked for a while and I understood where he was coming from and really what he needed, I thought there is definitely a role for me there." Could anyone besides Tyler Summitt have coaxed DeMoss back to college? "I don't know. I really don't know. This is bigger than a job. It's definitely a special situation," she said.

Tyler's mother taught him that a coach's staff is the most important part of a program, and he made the correct decisions when he started as a head coach. He hired DeMoss and added two assistants in Amber Smith, who played at Kentucky and was a graduate assistant for Tennessee, and Bernitha Johnson, who was a Lady Vols basketball manager. Mandy Miller, the head athletic trainer, was a graduate assistant at Tennessee under the direction of Moshak.

It wasn't thought that a Division I head coach would ever get as early a career start as Pat Summitt did, a job in 1974 that meant setting up the benches in the gym, sweeping the court, taping ankles, arranging for the officials to be there, washing uniforms, and driving the team van. She was also enrolled as a graduate student, in training for the 1976 Olympics and teaching classes at Tennessee. But Tyler had shown a knack for the game from an early age, one honed from watching hundreds of hours of film with his mother while still in high school. She never encouraged him to coach, but it was inevitable. Tyler was an honor roll student at an elite private school in Knoxville and could have entered any field following college. But he wanted to coach.

"He went to basketball school from infant on. And athletics department school because of everybody he was surrounded by," Moshak said. "He was being groomed, in a sense, without even knowing it because Pat was ready for him to not even be in coaching. When he was deciding between Tennessee and Vanderbilt, Pat came up to me and said, 'You know, I really hope he chooses Tennessee, not because I necessarily want him close to me, but if he really wants to coach, I don't want to pay for Vanderbilt tuition if he wants to be a coach.'"

DeMoss knows both mother and son perhaps as well as anyone. She was on the trip with Summitt when she went into labor during a recruiting trip to Macungie, Pennsylvania, to see Michelle Marciniak. She was in the delivery room with the rest of the coaching staff when Tyler entered the world.

Pat Summitt traveled to Louisiana to visit with her son and DeMoss and watch some games while he was there. Warlick also kept in touch with her longtime friend and teased her about working for Tyler. "When Tyler approached, she called me up and said, 'Am I crazy? Have I lost my mind?'" Warlick said. "I said, 'What does your gut tell you?'" The answer was to say yes. "There was an opportunity for me to give back to Pat, to give back to Louisiana Tech," DeMoss said. "That was where I had played. My family is here. I never thought I would go back to college. I thought I was going to finish out my career in the pros. But you never say never. You think you've got life planned out, and God kind of laughs at you." DeMoss, Summitt, and Warlick later chatted via FaceTime. "She told Pat, 'I forgot what it was like to build a program,'" Warlick said. "She said, 'Pat, I need you to come down here and help me.'"

Warlick stepped into Summitt's shoes at Tennessee, though Warlick likes to point out she had footprints to follow, not sneakers to fill. Warlick has restored a defensive mindset and vowed to recruit and win without compromising the principles taught by Summitt.

Warlick smiles and laughs when she talks about Summitt. "Pat still saw me as a daughter and a player," Warlick said. But she falls silent when asked to define Summitt's legacy, absorbing the enormity of the question. "Pat's legacy? When you think of her you, you think of championships. But I think of integrity, a woman who helped women succeed. She did everything in her power to say that women can do whatever the hell they want to do. Whether it's business, athletics, be a mother, everything she did was do not be held back because you're female. Leadership and teaching. She is the reason everyone is making the salaries they are making. TV. Pat empowered women to be better and to be the best they could ever be. And don't let any obstacle stop you. She showed that path to them."

Meshia Thomas was enriched by crossing paths with Summitt. A decision to leave Nashville and get on her feet in Knoxville—Thomas briefly needed YWCA housing and is an advocate for the agency now—led Thomas to walking beside the game's greatest coach. "She is awesome. She is an icon.

She is a woman so many of us can learn from day to day. She is the epitome of grace. If we could bottle her up, her grace, her style and dignity and just give it away, the world would definitely be a better place."

Cierra Burdick wanted more than one season with Summitt. "You want to be able to play under Pat as long as you can just because of the great coach that she is. The older players talked about her being a mother figure and that is the way I looked at her. I never questioned my loyalty to her. It was all worth it."

Taber Spani is a woman of tremendous faith. She summoned every bit of it to keep going when her head coach was diagnosed with dementia. Keep lacing up her basketball shoes. Keep leading her team. Keep praying for her coach. "It was difficult, and it was difficult because it was so unprecedented. The coaches and Pat were trying to figure out how to walk this out, and as players you were wanting to not just go all out for your team but there was the added pressure that we could be the last team. And then the national spotlight poured out on us that season and gave us the tremendous opportunity to showcase the Tennessee team and Pat.

"We just tried to go out and play, but it was difficult. It was new. Tragic and program changing. There are things you deal with constantly. Everyone will always remember that last season. Unprecedented is the word I would use. Honestly, as hard as it was, I am so privileged and blessed to be able to represent her for her last team."

Let's end it there. Pat Summitt would want the final word on her final season to come from a player.

AFTERWORD

In 2011, Pat Summitt was still coaching basketball. By early 2016, she had moved to assisted living. That is how fast early onset dementia can wreak havoc with someone's life—and those who love them.

On June 28, 2016, Summitt died from the devastating effects of the disease. While it was known that her condition had deteriorated, especially over the last year, the swiftness of Summitt's decline and subsequent death were startling.

In January 2014, a few months after signing the contract to write this book, I learned my own mother had Alzheimer's. As with anyone struggling to deal with this brutal disease, she forgets basic things and needs reminders of people in her past, including family members. But, for some reason, she had full recall that I was writing a book about Pat Summitt. When I called her at home in Washington, D.C., where she has lived since 1978, she would mention Summitt by name and ask how the book was coming together. The day before I received this manuscript in June 2016 for a final edit, I learned my mother had to be moved to a memory care center. My mother wrote her entire life, especially short stories, and read all the time, especially newspapers, books, poems, and magazines. Perhaps that is why the connection endured in her brain.

Every hour spent on this book seemed to have a dual purpose—tell the story of how the Lady Vols persevered under heartbreaking circumstances and also try to get it finished to present a copy to my mother while she could still read it.

Four seasons passed with Summitt serving in the role of head coach emeritus—one that diminished in duties over time due to her declining health—and with Holly Warlick leading the team.

Warlick has enjoyed considerable success: her teams have made three Elite Eight appearances and she has reached 100 career wins faster than almost any coach in the history of the sport. She has done so under unprecedented conditions as she watched her mentor, coach, and mother figure change from a dynamic force of nature on the basketball court to one compromised by a disease that spares no one from its ravaging effects.

Warlick also has been at the helm during a turbulent time at the University of Tennessee, marked by the dissolution of the women's athletics department; a contentious federal lawsuit claiming the university's culture enables sexual assaults by student-athletes, especially football players (which led the head coaches of all sports to hold a press conference in 2016 to rebut the accusations and was settled in July 2016 for $2.48 million); and the removal of the Lady Vols logo for all women's sports except basketball. That decision engendered such ill will and backlash that the Tennessee legislature got involved and a compromise was reached with the university that allows the other female athletes to wear a Lady Vols patch—if they choose—starting with the 2016 season. The Lady Vol proponents have vowed to continue the fight to restore the logo to all women's sports, especially after the death of Summitt.

Amid that environment, Warlick had to replace one of the sport's most iconic figures—and do so while maintaining Summitt's standards of excellence, especially with regard to recruiting. That meant no package deals, such as offering a scholarship to a sister to get the talented sibling or finding a spot on the staff for the parent of a coveted recruit. It also meant the teammate of a high school All-American player would not be offered a scholarship to help get the top recruit, only to yank the teammate's offer when the targeted player went elsewhere. While it is not against NCAA rules to do so, Summitt found such practices to be unethical. Her oft-repeated quote was: "Tennessee is not for everyone."

During a trying 2015–16 season in which the Lady Vol basketball team lost 13 regular-season games before the NCAA tourney, but still made it to the Elite Eight, Warlick had to press forward while being undermined within her own sport. A report out of Louisville, vehemently denied by Tennessee, said the University of Louisville's head coach had been approached by "boosters" about the Tennessee job, were it to come open. It was laughable and preposterous—there are no "boosters" who would have made contact like that—but the story had its day in the media due to the echo chamber of the Internet. When Louisville fell in the second round of the NCAA tourney—on its home court no less—it seemed like the appropriate ending.

The 2016 Women's Final Four featured only one No. 1 seed in perennial powerhouse University of Connecticut and three teams, Syracuse, Washington, and Oregon State, that were making their debuts on the game's biggest stage. Tennessee had beaten two of them, Oregon State and Syracuse, in the regular season. That level of parity is exactly what Summitt had envisioned for the sport, why she tirelessly promoted it, why she took her team all over the country to play, and why she agreed to a series in 1995 with the University of Connecticut team when Geno Auriemma had an upstart program that would go on to become a juggernaut. (Summitt ended the series in 2007 because she suspected serious recruiting shenanigans that she didn't expect from an elite coach. Warlick and Auriemma tried to restore the series in 2013, but Auriemma demanded an apology—another laughable and preposterous position—for Summitt's accusations, and Warlick rightfully refused. If the two programs ever meet in postseason, it will be an epic clash for the sport.)

Still, the standard of excellence for Tennessee is a Final Four and national championship—and Warlick knows it. The Lady Vols last appeared at the Final Four in 2007 and 2008 and won back-to-back national titles. Warlick wants nothing more than to get back, and Tennessee has come tantalizingly close with her at the helm.

In 2015, the Lady Vols played the postseason without senior center Isabelle Harrison (serious knee injury) and lost to Maryland one game short of the Final Four. In 2016, junior point guard Jordan Reynolds suffered a concussion in the Sweet 16 game and had to miss the Elite Eight matchup against Syracuse. Seniors Bashaara Graves and Andraya Carter had their hands broken in that same Sweet 16 game and played against Syracuse with soft casts that essentially reduced them to one-handed basketball players. They would have surgery a week later. Would Tennessee have won those games and made it to the Final Four if all players were healthy? There's no way to know for sure, but the Lady Vols would have relished being at full strength.

Cierra Burdick was a senior on the team that lost to Maryland in 2015. She went on to a professional career overseas and in the WNBA. After Burdick departed, the upcoming summer for the Lady Vols would include the switch to the incredibly popular Nike brand and a trip to Italy for a series of exhibition games. The seniors on the 2014–15 team were teased about missing it. But Burdick had the perfect reply.

"We played for Pat," Burdick said. "Nobody else can say that except the ones who came before us. We take honor in being the legacy class. When we talk about our experience at UT right now, five years down the line, ten years down the line, it will be one of the things that we talk about. We were the last class to play for Pat. We got to experience being coached by one of the greatest coaches to ever be. As time goes by, we'll appreciate it even more."

The most vexing question, however, is could Summitt have coached another year?

Summitt wanted one more season, especially so she could coach the final class that committed to her in Carter, Graves, and Jasmine Jones. She also wanted Tyler Summitt to join her on the sideline. In hindsight, he should have started on a much lower rung of the coaching ladder, such as a graduate assistant position for the Lady Vols. Getting a Division I assistant coach's position without any real experience and then becoming a head coach two years later clearly was too much too soon for him. While Tyler rightly was lauded for how he handled his mother's diagnosis at such a young age and his basketball acumen honed from years of watching film with his mother, he wasn't ready to carry the legacy of that name—and who could to be honest? He was also devastated by her illness, a sadness he kept deep inside. His downfall compounded an already crushing situation with his mother's disease. As F. Scott Fitzgerald wrote, "Show me a hero, and I'll write you a tragedy."

It is sometimes said that no one is bigger than the game. That adage crumbles when it comes to Summitt. She was Tennessee basketball. She was the reason for the eight championship banners, tens of thousands of fans in attendance, and multimillionaire coaching and TV contracts. She wanted to exit the court on her terms and didn't get the chance to do so.

Summitt deserved one last shot, but she never got to take it.

"Pat has brought so much attention to this disease for the greater good," Burdick said. "I was blessed to be a part of her story."

We all were. And we will all miss her.

PAT SUMMITT
(June 14, 1952–June 28, 2016)

ACKNOWLEDGMENTS

I have to open the acknowledgments with a thank you to Pat Summitt. Without her open book policy with the media throughout her coaching career, this book would not be possible. Summitt allowed the media access to every aspect of the Lady Vols program from practices to even film sessions at times. Because of her willingness to always help writers do their jobs better, I had a front-row seat for years to her program. It was the best basketball education I ever received.

I also want to thank all of the coaches and players who agreed to interviews for this book after the final season concluded: Holly Warlick, Dean Lockwood, Mickie DeMoss, Vicki Baugh, Glory Johnson, Meighan Simmons, Taber Spani, Cierra Burdick, Candace Parker, and Angie Bjorklund. Also, Summitt's son, Tyler; Meshia Thomas, Summitt's security detail; Jenny Moshak, the longtime chief of sports medicine for the Lady Vols; and the parents of Summitt's final three recruits: Keinya Graves, LaTrish Jones, Tyke Lhamon, and Jessica Lhamon. Thank you, too, to the entire 2011–12 team. All of the players were forthcoming with interviews during the final season and those have been captured in this book. Summitt's final three incoming recruits, Andraya Carter, Bashaara Graves, and Jasmine Jones, also wrote what it meant to be a Lady Vol before they arrived on campus, and those remarks were included, too.

Thanks also are extended to Scot Danforth of University of Tennessee Press, who believed in a first-time book author; Emily Huckabay, who helped guide me through the stages of the publishing process; Kelly Gray, book designer; Tom Post, publicist; and Debby Schriver, who was the initial reviewer and copy editor.

I also want to thank Cynthia Moxley and Alan Carmichael. I went to work as a writer/editor for their longtime communications firm, Moxley

Carmichael, shortly before signing the book contract. They both understood my passion for this book and sports and supported my extracurricular endeavors.

I also must thank Sally Jenkins, who wrote the definitive book on Summitt's life and career, *Sum It Up*, published in 2013. I reviewed the book for *InsideTennessee* and noted the final season, which was a chapter in the all-encompassing *Sum It Up*, was worth a book in itself. Jenkins contacted me and said: "You were there. You write it." So I did.

Finally, I thank my mother, Rosalie Cornelius. When I was a child, she turned off the television and sent me to the library. She told me the life I wanted would be found in books.

INDEX

Numbers in **bold** indicate photos.